Collins

need to know?

Food
Allergies

General editor:
Helen Stracey

Collins

First published in 2007 by Collins

an imprint of
HarperCollins Publishers
77–85 Fulham Palace Road
London W6 8JB

www.collins.co.uk

Collins is a registered trademark of HarperCollins Publishers Ltd

09   08   07
4   3   2   1

Text © HarperCollins Publishers, 2007

A catalogue record for this book is available from the British Library

General editor: Helen Stracey
Text: Karen Sullivan
Editor: Joanna Carreras
Designer: Bob Vickers
Series design: Mark Thomson
Artwork: Ome Design
Front and back cover photographs: © Getty Images

ISBN-10: 0-00-720160-5
ISBN-13: 978-0-007201-60-0

Colour reproduction by Printing Express Ltd, Hong Kong
Printed and bound by Printing Express Ltd, Hong Kong

Acknowledgments

The author would like to thank the staff at the Evelina Children's Hospital Allergy Clinic in London, including Gillian Dumont and Hasita Prinja, and Dr Adrian Morris of the Surrey Allergy Clinic, for providing a wealth of advice and information. Thanks also to Antoinette Savill for providing recipes, and to the Hospital for Sick Children in Toronto, Canada, for offering practical advice on weaning and breastfeeding. Allergy UK, The Anaphylaxis Campaign and British Society for Allergy and Clinical Immunology also helped a great deal with the facts and fine details. Thanks to Marcus, Eleanor and the other children who had their stories told.

Contents

Introduction 6

1 **Understanding food allergy** 9

2 **Foods that cause allergy** 23

3 **Identification** 69

4 **Managing your allergies** 99

5 **Allergic children** 129

6 **Allergic illness** 153

7 **Preventing allergies** 175

Want to know more? 188

Glossary 189

Index 190

Introduction

Food allergies have become headline news in the past few years, and many people have jumped on what has become a celebrity bandwagon that blames food allergies for the majority of common illnesses. The fact is that although food allergies and intolerance are on the increase, the number of true sufferers is still a small percentage of the population, and the largest numbers affected are children. For those sufferers, food can become an enemy, and even life-threatening in some cases.

Food allergies are still a relatively unknown science and diagnosis, and you may find that many conventional practitioners are reluctant to confirm that food is at the root of your health problems. What's more, testing is not fully accurate, which makes diagnosis even harder, and symptoms vary so much between different people that it's almost impossible to decide which are related to food and which may be a symptom of something else.

The good news is that our knowledge of food allergies is growing all the time, and new developments in technology, research methods, food production and diagnosis mean that things can only get better. Prevention of allergies is also a relatively new and exciting arm of allergy science, and we now know that there are many preventative measures you can take to reduce the risk of allergies, no matter how susceptible you or your family might be.

This book is for anyone who has ever worried about food allergies, intolerance or sensitivities of any nature. We will look at the main problem foods, and the likely reactions they may cause; we will help you choose a diet that is not only nutritious and delicious, but fun and able to be eaten with friends or at restaurants. included are delicious recipes, tips and ideas for eating out, the best ways to treat your symptoms, including treating life-threatening reactions, as well as the most up-to-date information on conventional and complementary approaches to food allergies.

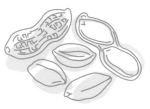

We examine the problem of allergies in children and adults, and work out the best way to provide optimum nutrition on a restricted diet. There are many ways to calculate whether food is your problem, and many of these start at home. This book is, in essence, your starter pack for assessing your allergies.

The most important message of this book is, however, that food allergies don't have to be a life sentence. Once you learn to read labels and adjust your diet accordingly, reactions can be a thing of the past, and you can go on to enjoy a variety of foods just like any other person. What's more, many allergies and intolerances can be outgrown. This book shows you how to get there – and how to enjoy the process of eating and living normally en route.

1 Understanding food allergy

Food allergies or food intolerance can trigger a host of unpleasant and in some cases frightening, violent and potentially fatal responses. Symptoms can express themselves all over the body and can range from swelling of the mouth, rashes and inflammation to wheezing and digestive problems. Currently there is no cure. Avoiding the offending food is the only viable solution and the key difficulty is identifying that food correctly. The good news is, however, that in many cases, scrupulously avoiding problem foods can mean that allergies are outgrown, particularly in childhood.

Allergy or intolerance: what is the difference?

Food allergies and intolerances are on the increase, particularly in the Western world and in children, yet they still remain a rarity in the developing world. Confusion, misinformation and controversy cloud the topic. Diagnosis can be vague, opinion can vary from one GP to another and many medical professionals are wary of making incorrect diagnoses.

The magnitude of the problem remains unknown, largely because the potential causes are numerous and can be difficult to identify. Many cases are mild enough to be undetected or may be misdiagnosed. Despite a dearth of statistics on the matter there is a consensus that true food allergy has increased significantly since the 1970s, particularly in the case of peanut allergy. Increased awareness and better understanding of allergies are insufficient to explain this increase. The rise in pollution levels, poor diet and certain immunizations have all been blamed for allergies in general, but the real reasons are still under investigation.

Food sensitivity

This is used as a general description to cover both allergy and intolerance. Accordingly food allergy or food intolerance are both types of food sensitivity. Some people can be 'sensitive' to certain foods or chemicals in foods, or they can become sensitive at certain times of their life – for example, after illness, during a menstrual cycle, after a course of

did you know?

In industrialized, highly developed communities, up to 20 per cent of the population experience adverse reactions to food and claim to be allergic to certain foods. However, estimates suggest that no more than five to eight per cent of children and one to two per cent of adults are affected by food allergy/intolerance and that less than one per cent of adults and one to two per cent of children are truly allergic to food.

antibiotics, during pregnancy, in periods of stress or emotional problems and after 'overeating' a specific food – but this does not necessarily mean they have a true food allergy or a definite pattern of intolerance.

Food aversion

This is not an allergy as such, but more of a psychological condition. It relates to a situation where a person strongly dislikes a food and believes that a food produces a particular reaction in them. Aversion usually stems from foods that are associated with sickness, nausea or gastrointestinal discomfort. So, in essence, a bad experience with food in one's childhood can lead to aversion in later life and the belief that it causes symptoms. Sometimes the associated symptoms are similar to those resulting from intolerances, which can potentially lead to misdiagnosis. Interestingly, however, many children and seriously allergic people have a natural aversion to foods that they are genuinely allergic to – some experts believe that this is one of the body's natural defence mechanisms.

Allergy or intolerance?

It is often very difficult to determine whether you have a food allergy or a food intolerance. The dividing line is so blurred. Many people mistakenly believe they have a food allergy when in fact they have food intolerance. One way to test this is that if you suffer from an intolerance you will usually be able to eat small amounts of problem foods without a reaction. In contrast, if you have a true food allergy, even a tiny amount of the food may trigger a serious allergic reaction. Symptoms of an allergy to any particular food also tend to appear much more quickly than the symptoms of an intolerance.

Food allergy

A food allergy involves the body's immune (defence) system and is a reaction that occurs when the body's immune system overreacts to a normally harmless substance, known as an allergen. This can cause an immediate and sometimes a severe reaction – for example, irritation, disability and, in the extreme, death from anaphylaxis (see pages 101-102). In a true food allergy, the immune system produces antibodies and histamine in response to the specific food. The next time you eat even the smallest amount of that food the antibodies sense it and signal your immune system again to release histamine and other chemicals into your blood stream. It is this reaction by the body that causes symptoms. It is common for children to grow out of a food allergy, particularly allergies to eggs, wheat and cow's milk. However, people with allergies to peanuts, nuts, fish and shellfish normally have the condition for life, even if they scrupulously avoid the food in question. Tests are available to test allergies that involve the immune response (see pages 77-79), but these are not clear cut. Positive tests do not necessarily imply a food allergy so a proper interpretation of results is necessary.

Food intolerance

A food intolerance describes an unpleasant reaction to an offending food. It is often triggered by foods that are both craved and eaten frequently. The jury is still out as to whether it involves the immune system, but as antibodies are not normally produced against the problem foods, it would seem that symptoms occur without the help of the immune

must know

Anaphylaxis

Pronounced anna-full-axis or sometimes called anaphylactic shock, this applies to the most severe allergic reaction, which can be potentially life threatening. Any food can cause anaphylaxis in susceptible people, if the allergy is severe. Reactions tend to become worse with subsequent exposure to problem foods.

system. The reaction and symptoms can be much more vague and slower to take effect; sometimes it can take from hours to days for symptoms to surface, making diagnosis difficult. The only reliable way to diagnose a food intolerance is to exclude completely the offending food/s to see if symptoms improve. If they do then the food should be reintroduced slowly to see if symptoms reappear. Symptoms can affect any part of the body, can be varied and are generally not life threatening. However, if you continue to eat a food to which you are intolerant, it could make you feel ill or affect your long-term health.

Intolerances may well disappear if the food is not eaten for a few months, but they tend to recur if ever the food is eaten regularly again. Food intolerances can occur for a variety of reasons including:

Non-allergic histamine release Foods such as shellfish or strawberries can trigger the release of histamine (also released in true allergic reactions) and produce signs very similar to an allergy. Headaches, swelling, urticaria (nettle rash or hives), vomiting and diarrhoea are all common reactions. Foods with high histamine levels can produce similar signs (see pharmacological reactions below).

Metabolic defects The most common problem is lactose intolerance. A deficiency in lactase, the enzyme responsible for digesting lactose in milk causes a reduction in the body's ability to digest lactose in all dairy products and results in an intolerance to milk. This kind of intolerance is more widespread in certain populations. For example, it affects between 50 and 90 per cent of people of

> **must know**
>
> **Coeliac disease**
> This is a gut intolerance to gluten, a protein found in wheat and rye, and to similar proteins found in barley. The intolerance is permanent and treatment is by complete and lifelong exclusion of gluten from the diet. Coeliac disease is thought to be an abnormal immunological response rather than a lack of certain digestive enzymes. It is not considered to be a food allergy in the true sense of the definition.

Indian and Afro-Caribbean origin but only about 15 per cent of the Caucasian population. The percentage of sufferers in the UK is therefore quite low. There is some evidence, however, to suggest that lactose intolerance is increasing in the West – possibly because the high levels of dairy produce in our diet require high levels of lactase to digest them, and, as we age, most people's lactase production declines. Furthermore, some experts believe that because inter-race marriages are much more common now, mixed-race children may carry the problematic genes.

Pharmacological reactions Some food substances can act like drugs particularly if taken in large quantities. The most familiar of these substances is caffeine, found in tea, coffee, chocolate and cola drinks. A large intake of caffeine can cause tremors, migraines and palpitations.

Other pharmacologically active substances found in food include the vasoactive amines (see must know box): histamine, tyramine, tryptamine and serotonin. These are powerful vasoconstrictors capable of producing in susceptible people symptoms such as urticaria (nettle rash or hives), facial flushing and headaches, nausea and giddiness. Tyramine can trigger migraine in some people. These vasoactive amines are present in many foods such as red wine, chocolate, cheese (especially if mature), fermented products such as blue cheese, sauerkraut and fermented soya products, yeast extracts, fish particularly if unfresh, pickles, microbially contaminated foods, some fruits such as avocados, citrus foods and bananas. The

must know

Vasoactive amines

These are normally deactivated in the body by the enzyme monoamine oxidase (MAO). People taking MAO-A inhibitor drugs (antidepressants) must avoid high intakes of foods high in vasoactive amines as they will slow the breakdown of these amines and lead to a dangerous rise in blood pressure.

word 'vasoactive' simply means that a substance causes the blood vessels to constrict *or* dilate – and this causes symptoms, such as flushing, palpitations, headaches and giddiness.

Monosodium glutamate (MSG) Commonly found in Chinese food and as a flavour enhancer. High amounts can cause flushing, headache and abdominal symptoms and may even mimic the symptoms of a heart attack with chest pain radiating to both arms and general weakness and palpitations.

Food intolerance of unknown origin Reactions can be provoked by many foods and food products for which the reasons are vague. They may or may not be allergic reactions. Food additives, particularly tartrazine and sodium benzoate, can provoke urticaria, rhinitis (inflammation of mucus membrane in the nose) and asthma. Yeast products can provoke several reactions in some people, particularly skin disorders.

must know

Allergic reactions
These are usually immediate, or occur at least within 72 hours of eating a particular food; they can be provoked by the tiniest amount. Food intolerance reactions tend to be much slower and are provoked by much larger quantities of food.

The allergic reaction

Our immune system plays an essential role in our bodies. It protects us from harmful foreign invaders such as viruses and bacteria that might otherwise cause illness. It produces a range of defences called antibodies, to fight off any invaders. Familiar signs of this fight in the body include swelling, redness and fever, all healthy signs that your immune system is working.

must know

Antibody: an immune cell that circulates in the bloodstream ready to destroy any substance (bacteria, toxin, dietary protein) that may enter the body.
IgE: Immunoglobulin E. A specific antibody associated with food allergies. Other antibodies and different types of immune reaction may also be involved.

In an allergic person the system recognizes harmless substances such as food and pollen as invaders (allergens) and attempts to fight them off. Once the system decides that a particular food is harmful it creates a specific antibody to it, IgE (immunogoblin E), which sticks to the surface of mast cells (specialist immune cells which contain histamine – the chemical released by the body in response to an allergic reaction). This is why you won't necessarily have a reaction the first time a particular food is eaten as the body needs to become sensitized to it.

So the next time you eat that food, the IgE antibody recognizes the invader and triggers the release of massive amounts of chemicals such as histamine from the mast cells. These cause the unpleasant symptoms such as rashes, inflammation or wheezing that are often associated with an allergic reaction. In rare and extreme cases a mild response can develop into a severe allergic reaction leading to what is known as an anaphylactic shock and possible death. Blood vessels dilate and the heart and lungs cease to function properly. Thankfully most allergic reactions are not this severe.

Foods that can cause common allergies/intolerances

Cow's milk *

Eggs*

Soya*

Wheat *

Peanuts*

Tree nuts* (Brazil nuts, almonds, hazelnuts) and sesame seeds

Fish*

Shellfish*

Chocolate

Caffeine

Wine

Some food additives

* the top eight foods to cause food allergy

Eight foods account for 90 per cent of all allergic reactions: cow's milk, eggs, soya, wheat, peanuts, tree nuts, fish and shellfish. Peanuts are the leading cause of severe allergic reactions, followed by shellfish, fish, tree nuts and eggs. It is important to remember, however, that *any* food can cause an allergic reaction, or a food intolerance, in susceptible people. See also Chapter Two.

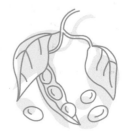

must know

Allergy and age
A food allergy can develop at any age, although it occurs in a smaller percentage of adults. Three to seven per cent of children will have a food allergy diagnosed before their third birthday, but it often disappears before adulthood.

Signs and symptoms

Signs and symptoms of food allergy or intolerance are not clear cut, except in the case of anaphylaxis. Allergies can affect the whole body and common symptoms typically include the following:

Head: headaches or migraine, loss of concentration

Eyes: itching, redness, watering, swelling

Ears: itching, deafness, glue ear, tinnitus (ringing in the ears)

Nose: sneezing and constant runny nose (perennial rhinitis), conjestion, itching

Sinuses: blockages, infection, pain

Mouth: swollen tongue, inflammation or ulcers, burning sensation

Larynx: swelling of the voicebox

Lungs: wheezing, coughing and shortness of breath (asthma), feeling of tightness, 'whistling' sound when breathing, congestion

Skin: itchy rashes (urticaria - nettle rash or hives) and dry flaky skin (eczema), dermatitis, rashes around the mouth and chin

Stomach & bowel: an uncomfortable bloated feeling, pain, diarrhoea, vomiting, flatulence (wind), itchy bottom, cramping, constipation

General: lethargy, flu-like aches and pains, fatigue, irritability

Who is at risk?

Although much is still unknown about allergies, we do know that certain groups of people are more susceptible. The diagnosis of allergy or intolerance to food is much more likely if any of these characteristics fit you or your background.

Atopy/heredity

Some families have an inherited tendency to develop allergies as a result of some slight change to a gene that is linked to production of immunogloblin E (IgE). This tendency is known as 'atopy', and it is more likely that someone from an atopic family will develop an allergy at some point in their lives. The type of allergy may take a different form and people who are allergic to some foods may also be allergic to other environmental factors, such as house dust, animal fur and pollen. Being atopic is strongly associated with allergic disease in the form of asthma, eczema and hay fever and it increases the risk of food allergy.

If you have one parent that suffers from food allergy or intolerance you have a 20 to 30 per cent chance of being allergic to something yourself although not necessarily the same allergy that affects your parent. If both parents are affected, the risk climbs to 40 to 60 per cent. However, a third of children with allergies are born to parents who are not aware of any allergic symptoms in themselves.

Other influences

Studies show that the more people are exposed to infections the less likely they are to develop

> **did you know?**
>
> A 2006 study found that avoiding the use of antibiotics and fever-reducers can reduce the risk of allergic disease, such as food allergies, eczema and asthma, in young children. Austrian scientist and philosopher Rudolf Steiner developed the 'anthroposophic' lifestyle in which health is a combination of mind, body and spiritual balance; his followers integrate modern medicine with alternative treatments. The study concluded that early use of antibiotics and fever reducers, and the measles, mumps and rubella vaccination, were associated with increased risks of several allergic symptoms and doctor's diagnoses.

must know

Allergic illnesses
It is claimed that food allergy and intolerance play a role in the development of the following:
- Asthma
- Eczema
- Irritable bowel syndrome
- Migraine
- Hyperactivity and behavioural disorders
- Chronic diseases – rheumatoid arthritis, chronic fatigue syndrome, depression, otitis media (inflammation of the middle ear)

See Chapter Six for further information.

allergies. Younger siblings and children who start nursery very early have been shown to suffer less from allergies than first or only children; this is because they come into more contact with infections from an earlier age.

Why are allergies increasing?

Reasons for the increase in allergies is still being debated and may be a consequence of a number of factors: modern living conditions, poor diet, smaller families, immunization, air pollution, greater use of chemicals and antibiotics and a more stressful lifestyle. There is some evidence to suggest that the switch to a more processed diet is to blame: processed food provides a more sterile diet with fewer natural antioxidants and natural vitamins, which are natural protectors against disease including allergic disease. What is more, they tend to be full of chemicals used in the manufacturing process, as well as additives and preservatives. All of these put a strain on the body, which can affect the immune response.

It is often the case that a food that is eaten more frequently in a particular country becomes the offending cause of allergy in that location. For example, in Sweden, more people are susceptible to fish allergies; in the UK it is wheat; and in the USA people are often allergic to maize (corn).

Growing out of it

Whether or not you grow out of your allergy depends on your age and your family history. For example, babies often outgrow moderate or mild food allergies but the longer they have the allergy, and the stronger the family history, the less likely they are to do so. Allergies that develop in adulthood rarely disappear completely, although they may improve with time. Similarly, food intolerances may also disappear to some degree, following a strict period of elimination.

want to know more?

For some of the ways you can prevent allergies from developing, see Chapter Seven.

AllergyUK (www.allergyuk.org) has a helpline that operates from 9-5 pm Monday to Friday. Staff can deal with a wide range of questions on food allergies, intolerance and any other allergic illness, including finding your nearest allergy clinic or specialist consultant. They can also give advice on dealing with symptoms and on products that may be beneficial. Call 01322 619898, or visit the website, which has a wealth of helpful information.

Dr Adrian Morris of the Surrey Allergy Clinic and BBC Health Online explains common allergies and their treatment on www.allergy-clinic.co.uk.

Action Against Allergy can supply information packs and leaflets on a wide range of subjects, including non-allergenic products and details of your nearest allergy clinic. Visit www.actionagainstallergy.co.uk or phone 020 8892 4949.

2 Foods that cause allergy

In reality, any food has the potential to cause allergic symptoms in susceptible people, so no single food can be ruled out. We do know, however, that eight main foods are responsible for some 90 per cent of food allergies, and a handful of other foods are commonly implicated. Let's look at the most common offenders, where they are found, and the symptoms they produce.

Cow's milk

There are two main problems with cow's milk. One involves the sugar in milk (lactose), which causes lactose intolerance. The other involves the protein in milk, which tends to be at the root of a true cow's milk allergy. Symptoms tend to differ between these two conditions, but it's often hard to distinguish which is at the root of the reactions.

Cow's milk is one of the most common food allergies in children (see page 133), perhaps because it is usually the first foreign protein that they encounter. While cow's milk allergies are becoming increasingly common in babies (some studies show that up to seven and a half per cent of infants are affected), a large majority of allergic children outgrow them before their seventh birthday. Unfortunately, lactose intolerance is rarely outgrown, and often becomes worse as we become older.

Although it may seem obvious, a milk allergy is an allergy to *all* dairy products, so cheese, milk, yoghurt, butter, milk-based puddings and any other foods that contain milk or milk products will not be tolerated. In the case of lactose intolerance, some dairy produce – particularly yoghurts – can be successfully introduced into the diet, and the amount tolerated will differ between individuals.

Not all milks are the same as cow's milk, and a cow's milk allergy does not necessarily mean that you are allergic to all animal milks. Some cow's milk allergy sufferers (recent studies show around 40 per cent) can tolerate goat's and sheep's milk and foods that contain them, largely because the protein make-up is slightly different. But it's worth noting that goat's or sheep's milk will not be tolerated by lactose intolerant individuals, because all milks contain lactose, including breastmilk. The symptoms differ between the two conditions: lactose intolerance and allergy.

Lactose intolerance

Lactose is the main sugar found in milk (and therefore all dairy products, including breast milk and standard milk formulas for infants). When you are lactose intolerant, it simply means that you are unable to digest this type of sugar, largely because of a shortage of a digestive enzyme called lactase, which is normally produced in the small intestine. Lactase is responsible for breaking down milk sugar in order that it can be absorbed into the blood stream. When there is not enough lactase available to digest lactose, painful gastrointestinal symptoms result. Most commonly, these include diarrhoea, bloating, cramps, gas and nausea.

did you know?

People who suffer from cow's milk allergy will often go on to experience other allergies. For example, half of all sufferers will develop an allergy to other food proteins such as egg, soya or peanuts, and between 50 and 80 per cent will develop an allergy to one or more 'inhalant' allergens, such as grass pollens, dust mites, or animal dander. There is also a higher risk of developing other allergic conditions, such as asthma or eczema.

Symptoms do vary in severity, depending on how intolerant you are or, in other words, how much lactase is being produced in the intestine. It also depends on how much lactose is consumed.

There is undoubtedly an ethnic link to this condition, and Westernized Africans and South-east Asians, some Eastern Europeans and even some Mediterranean populations (and their descendants) tend to be one of the hardest hit, with as many as 90 per cent suffering. In all people, however, lactase is produced in decreasing quantities after the age of about two years, but symptoms may not manifest themselves until much later in life.

A tiny percentage of babies are actually born without the ability to produce lactase, and this makes feeding difficult. Other causes include digestive disorders (such as diarrhoea), injuries to the small intestine, and even repeated courses of antibiotics, which destroy the healthy intestinal bacteria (known as flora) and upset the intestine's ability to produce this enzyme. However, this is usually only a short-term problem and can be resolved.

There are a variety of different tests used to diagnose this condition, including breath tests, stool acidity and blood tests (see page 79). Apart from stool acidity tests, these are not recommended for children. If symptoms present themselves, it's commonly agreed that withdrawal of all dairy produce is the best course of action. Many children later find that they can reintroduce small quantities of dairy produce into their diets, but others experience discomfort throughout their lives. In some cases, lactose intolerance can become apparent in later life, although this is not usual.

Young children with lactase deficiency should not eat any foods containing lactose. Older children and adults can often manage small quantities, but acceptable levels will differ. It's really just a question of trying out different foods to ascertain which cause the most problems.

It is also possible to purchase lactase enzymes at some chemists and health food shops, and these come in a variety of different forms. Drops, for example, can be added to milk and left for 24 hours, after which the lactose content is reduced significantly. Others include chewable tablets, which are taken just before any food that contains lactose. It's also worth looking out for lactose-reduced dairy products (in particular, milk and yoghurt) which contain the same levels of nutrients as brands with the normal levels of lactose. Some sufferers can tolerate yoghurt as the lactose has been fermented by bacteria; hard cheese is naturally low in lactose and is also often well tolerated. It is very important to try to include some cheese, yoghurt and lactose-reduced milk in your diet, as it is an excellent source of calcium and vitamins.

Remember, all animal milks contain lactose, so substituting goat's or sheep's milk will not have any effect.

Milk allergy

A milk allergy is different to lactose intolerance. Instead of being unable to digest lactose, someone suffering from a milk allergy has a reaction to the *protein* in milk. It's also possible to be sensitive to or intolerant of the proteins in milk, as well as being

must know
Hidden lactose
Lactose is added to many foods as a natural sweetener, so anyone suffering from an intolerance should be aware of the types of foods in which it appears. It's very easy to absorb more than you can handle, so take time to read labels, and watch out for the following foods:
• breads, cakes, pastries, biscuits
• soups
• sweets, chocolate bars
• margarines
• processed cereals and breakfast cereals
• salad dressings
Lactose is also used in a number of prescription drugs and over-the-counter medicines, so check with your pharmacist.

lactose intolerant. In these circumstances, it's best to avoid all dairy produce completely.

The two main protein components are whey and casein, and you may be allergic to either or both. The casein is the curd that forms when milk is left to sour, and the whey is the watery liquid that is left after the curd is removed. Whey proteins are less allergenic than casein proteins.

Whey (which makes up about 20 per cent of milk) contains mainly alpha-lactalbumin and beta-lactaglobulin and is most likely to produce the IgE-antibodies (Immunoglobulin E – see page 16) and causes the most clinical problems. These IgE-antibodies can be tested for in the blood, and by skin prick testing (see page 77). The whey proteins are altered by high heat, and so some sufferers may be able to tolerate evaporated, boiled or sterilized (UHT) milk and milk powder.

Casein is not affected by heat, so anyone who is allergic to casein will probably react to all types of milk and milk products – even cheese, as casein is the part of the milk used to make cheese. The harder the cheese, the more casein is formed.

The degree to which you are allergic will vary. There are three main types of reactions. They can occur immediately, or start several hours or even days after the intake of moderate to large amounts of cow's milk. In some sufferers, even a tiny amount will cause a reaction.

Type 1 - *Immediate* symptoms start within minutes of eating or drinking small amounts of cow's milk or dairy products. These usually include skin problems, eczema, urticaria (hives), as well as respiratory symptoms such as a runny nose or wheezing. Many people will experience

watch out!

Symptoms in babies and children indicating a possible milk allergy
- excessive colic
- recurrent diarrhoea
- vomiting, abdominal pain
- rash, hives and eczema
- chronic runny nose
- nasal stuffiness
- recurrent bronchitis
- recurrent 'colds' and sinusitis
- ear infections
- coughing
- irritability
- failure to thrive (in infants)

immediate gastro-intestinal symptoms, such as vomiting and diarrhoea. In some sufferers this immediate reaction can be dangerous or even life threatening.

Type 2 - *Intermediate* symptoms start between one and 24 hours after a modest intake of cow's milk. Sufferers will usually experience vomiting or diarrhoea, and other gastrointestinal problems.

Type 3 - *Late* symptoms develop between one and five days after taking in large quantities of cow's milk. Symptoms include diarrhoea, with or without respiratory or skin reactions.

Much the same symptoms will appear in children and babies, but there are a few other things to look out for (see page 183-84).

Cow's milk and nutrition

The main nutrients contained in milk and other dairy products include protein, lots of calcium, and some B vitamins. Full-fat milk also contains vitamins A, D and E. All round, it's a good nutritious fast food, but it is not essential, despite advertisements to the contrary. If you cut out milk you will need to ensure that you make up for the lost nutrients; in particular, calcium, which can be hard to replace (particularly in children, who tend to resist vegetables and fish, and in multiple allergy sufferers, who may also be allergic to fish and seeds).

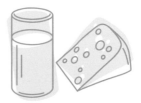

Hidden milk protein

Milk is used in a wide variety of different foods, and listed on the label under various names. It's crucial that you take time to read the labels to ensure that milk isn't an extra hidden ingredient. You need to look out for:

butter
artificial butter flavour
butter solids/fat
caramel colour
caramel flavouring
casein
caseinate
ammonium caseinate
calcium caseinate
hydrolyzed casein
iron caseinate
magnesium caseinate
potassium caseinate
rennet casein
sodium caseinate
sodium caseinate solids
zinc caseinate
cheese
cream
curds
high protein flour
lactalbumin
lactalbumin phosphate
lactoferrin

lactoglobulin
lactose
margarine
milk
buttermilk
milk derivative
milk fat
milk protein
milk solids
skimmed milk
cottage cheese
powdered milk
dried milk
dry milk solids
sour milk solids
hydrolyzed milk protein
sour cream solids
whey
delactosed whey
demineralized whey
whey protein concentrate
whey powder
yoghurt

Be aware that 'non-dairy' products may contain casein. Anything that has the words 'whey', 'casein', 'caseinate', 'lactalbumin' or lactose in the name will be problematic.

Milk proteins are also found in custard, many biscuits, cakes and breads, most chocolates and some brands of tinned tuna. Even sausages and cured meats, such as hams, may contain milk products. They are obviously found in yoghurts, fromage frais, many dips, crème fraîche, and white/bechamel sauces.

Nutrient sources

- Leafy green vegetables are a good source of calcium, in particular sprouting broccoli, watercress and kale, and fish with soft, edible bones, such as salmon (tinned is fine). Whitebait and sardines are also an excellent option. Almonds are also high in calcium as are soya bean curd and sesame seeds. Recent research shows that yoghurt may be a good source of calcium for many people with lactose intolerance, although it is fairly high in lactose. It appears that the bacterial cultures used in making yoghurt produce some of the lactase enzyme required for proper digestion. It also helps to improve the health of the intestine, which ensures normal function and better absorption of nutrients.
- Vitamin A is also found in most brightly coloured vegetables (as beta-carotene) and in meats, eggs, liver and fish liver oil.
- Vitamin D is also found in eggs, fish liver oils, vegan margarines and most oily fish. The very best source of vitamin D is, of course, sunlight.
- Soya, vegetable oils, leafy green vegetables and eggs will also provide adequate amounts of vitamin E.

did you know?

Milk allergy almost always presents in the first year of life, soon after the introduction of cow's milk or cow's milk-based infant formula, and usually resolves by school age. Most infants with cow's milk allergy develop gastrointestinal symptoms (about 60 per cent), approximately 50 to 70 per cent develop skin problems, and some 33 per cent will have respiratory symptoms.

must know

Calcium

This is the most important nutrient that milk and milk products provide. If you do not get enough in your diet, a calcium supplement may be the best source – particularly for teenagers and breastfeeding mothers.

Eggs

Egg allergy is one of the most common causes of food allergies in babies and young children, although studies show that it is almost always outgrown (in about 80 per cent of cases) by the age of five.

must know

Avoid all bird's eggs, as chicken's eggs are not the only culprits.
To add variety to your diet you can substitute eggs in recipes with egg replacers (see page 120). Or buy vegan food – this is always egg free.

Foods containing egg

Unfortunately, eggs are found in a huge number of products, including baked goods, sauces, breaded meats, cereals, flours, sweets, biscuits, custards, noodles, desserts, fondants, some processed meats, ice cream, pasta, malted drinks, mayonnaise, meringues, soups, salad dressings, sausages, pancakes, egg noodles and even some wines. Many breads and baked goods are brushed with egg to provide an attractive finish. Even worse, many cosmetics, including shampoos, contain egg proteins, so be sure to read the labels carefully.

Proteins

Once again, proteins are at the root of this allergy. The main proteins responsible for egg allergies are present in the egg white, but some proteins are found in the yolk; both can induce allergy. Cooking denatures many of the egg proteins, which explains why some people can eat cooked eggs, but react to raw eggs – in homemade mayonnaise, for example.

Most egg-allergic children are allergic to proteins in the egg white, although some are allergic to the yolk. There are three yolk proteins that tend to cause problems, but allergies to these are less common in

Eggs are listed under a multitude of different terms, and egg-allergic or -sensitive people will need to be aware of them all. Watch out for:

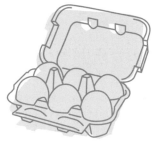

- albumin
- dried egg
- egg
- egg white
- egg yolk
- egg powder/powdered egg
- egg solids
- egg substitutes
- globulin
- pasteurized egg
- frozen egg
- ovalbumin
- ovumucin, ovomucoid, ovoglobulin, ovotransferrin
- vitellin, livetin, ovovitelia, ovovitellin

Very rarely, lecithin may also be made with egg yolks.

It is also important to be aware that children who are highly allergic to egg can suffer a mild reaction from eggs being fried in the same room, touching someone who has been in contact with raw eggs, or even sitting close to someone who is eating egg.

children. Eggs from birds other than hens can cause an allergy reaction in children with a significant hen's egg allergy, as the proteins are the same.

In some children, the reaction is triggered by inhaled bird antigens – a condition known as bird-egg syndrome. Interestingly, egg allergies can also be seasonal. Children who suffer from some types of hay fever may cross-react with eggs when some pollens are in season.

Most egg allergy reactions, including severe reactions, occur between six and 15 months of age, when egg is given for the first time. At this stage, the child is often very highly sensitized because the allergy has not been appreciated and there has been contact with little bits of protein through breast milk or in biscuits or other foods in the diet.

The symptoms associated with egg allergy include allergic rhinitis, asthma, dermatitis, diarrhoea, gastrointestinal symptoms, hives, nausea, vomiting, wheezing and, in some cases, anaphylaxis

must know

Mild allergy
If your egg allergy is mild, perhaps only causing a flare-up of eczema or itching, you may be able to tolerate small traces of egg in cooked goods, such as breads, cakes and biscuits.

(see page 101). Egg allergy is the most common food hypersensitivity in children with eczema.

Research indicates that egg allergy is less common in adults (more commonly a culprit of food intolerance), although highly allergic adults may suffer some nausea or flaring of eczema after eating egg that is a major ingredient in food. However, according to Robert Loblay, from the Allergy Unit at RPA Hospital in Australia, this doesn't happen very often as those with an egg allergy tend to have a natural aversion to eating eggs. Moreover, most egg-allergic adults can eat egg if it is a minor ingredient in a food.

Eggs and nutrition

Eggs are a good source of first-class protein, and contain B-vitamins (especially B1) as well as many other nutrients, including zinc, vitamins A, D and E, and lecithin, a mineral that is necessary for the metabolic processes of the body.

While eggs are not essential, you will need to ensure that you get protein from other sources, such as pulses, wholegrains, meat and fish, seeds, soya, nuts and dairy produce. Multiple allergies can often rule many of these foods out, so you will need the help of a dietitian to make sure your needs are being met. A good multi-vitamin and mineral supplement, as well as a diet that is rich in fresh fruit and vegetables, will supply adequate vitamins and minerals.

watch out!

The MMR injection is normally cultured on egg. Anaphylactic reactions to the MMR have been reported, but they are very rare. In any case, It is probable that in those instances, a component other than egg was responsible. If there are any concerns, the vaccination should be given to the child as an outpatient in a paediatric department with full resuscitation equipment available. Normally a test dose is given before the full dose.

Soya

Soya (also called soy) allergy is more common in children than in adults and occurs in between five and 30 per cent of all people – although it is more likely to be a cause of food intolerance than true allergy.

Hidden ingredients

Ingredients that can suggest soya content:
- gum arabic/guar gum
- soy panthenol
- bulking agent
- carob
- soy protein isolate or concentrate
- emulsifier
- soya sauce
- hydrolyzed vegetable protein (HVP)
- soybean
- lecithin
- soybean oil
- miso starch
- MSG (monosodium glutamate)
- textured vegetable protein (TVP)
- protein thickener/extender
- tofu (soya bean curd)
- soya flour
- soya milk/yoghurt/ cheese
- soya nuts
- vegetable starch/ gum/protein/broth

Interestingly, research shows that if you suffer from a cow's milk allergy, you are also more likely to suffer from a soya allergy; and if you suffer from a soya allergy, you are likely to be allergic to one or more foods.

An allergy to soya simply means an adverse reaction to one or more of the proteins in soya, and we know that there are at least five. These allergic reactions may be caused by eating foods containing soya, or by inhaling soya dust. Breastfed babies may also suffer from soya allergies as a result of soya protein passing through the breastmilk.

It is unknown whether soya lecithin, soya margarine or soya oil contain sufficient protein to provoke allergic reactions. In some studies those with soya allergy could tolerate small amounts of soya oil, lecithin and margarine, but in other studies patients could not.

It's also worth noting that if you are allergic to soya beans, you may also be allergic to foods in the same family, which share a similar protein structure. Soya beans are legumes (pulses), so caution should be taken when eating other legumes, such as green peas, broad beans (lima beans), and chick peas.

The problem with a soya allergy is that it is virtually impossible to eliminate soya completely from the diet, as it is 'hidden' in so many foods. Product labelling laws state that all ingredients must be listed on the label of any food. However, soya is often used to influence the manufacturing process, or to increase the protein level in foods, and may be hidden *within* other ingredients on the product's label. For example, if margarine is added to a food product, it will be listed as such, but soya present in the margarine itself will not be listed on the ingredients panel. Also, certain food additives are manufactured from the soya bean and may retain the allergic potential (allergenicity). These include soya lecithin and soya emulsifier. So anyone with a soya allergy should aim for a soya-restricted diet, as complete elimination is never possible. It is used, simply, in far too many foods and processes.

The most common symptoms include vomiting, diarrhoea, abdominal cramps, itching of the skin, hives (urticaria), facial swelling and eczema. Asthma, hay fever, shortness of breath and swelling of the throat have also been noted, and, in rare cases, anaphylaxis (see page 101) can occur. Vomiting and coughing and wheezing usually occur within two hours of ingestion with more severe reactions, such as gastrointestinal symptoms, following in 24 to 48 hours.

Soya and nutrition

Soya can be an essential source of protein for vegetarians and vegans; however, it is not the only source. If tolerated, nuts, seeds, eggs (not for vegans), pulses and dairy produce are all good sources of protein. Quorn may also be useful.

Soya in foods

Foods that may contain soya protein include:
- baby foods/formula
- baked goods
- margarine
- meat products (sausage, cold meats, etc., particularly vegetarian substitutes)
- breakfast cereals/muesli
- burgers
- pies
- butter substitutes
- salad dressings
- tinned meat or fish
- sauces (e.g. Worcestershire, sweet and sour, HP, Teriyaki)
- tinned or packaged soups
- seasoned salt
- Chinese food
- snack bars
- chocolate
- cooking oils
- pasta products
- soya sauce
- soya sprouts
- gravy powders
- hot dogs
- stock cubes (bouillon)
- ice-cream
- tofu

Wheat

It is possible to be allergic to the proteins in wheat and/or intolerant or simply sensitive to wheat itself. The enthusiasm for wholegrains and dietary fibre over the past decade has lead to a trend in overeating grains – in particular, wheat.

Many cases of intolerance and sensitivity are due more to overeating than a true allergy. However, true allergies do exist, particularly in children and adults who suffer from multiple allergies.

Wheat allergy refers specifically to adverse reactions involving immunoglobulin E (IgE) antibodies to one or more protein elements of wheat, including albumin, globulin, gliadin and glutenin (gluten). The majority of IgE-mediated reactions to wheat involve the albumin and globulin fractions. Gliadin and gluten may also induce IgE-mediated reactions although rarely.

Gluten is also found in other cereal grains, such as rye, oats and barley. Those who suffer from coeliac disease or 'coeliac sprue' suffer from a permanent, adverse reaction to gluten, and will not lose their sensitivity to this substance. The only treatment is lifelong restriction of gluten – and that means to any of the grains that contain it.

However, those who have a wheat allergy (an immune-mediated response to wheat protein), must avoid only wheat. Confusing, it is, but there are differences between the gluten found in the various grains, and studies show that wheat-allergic people can normally eat other gluten-containing grains without any problem. Most wheat-allergic children outgrow the allergy.

did you know?

The Coeliac Society (www.coeliac.co.uk) publishes a comprehensive list of manufactured products that are gluten-free on an annual basis; regular updates appear on its website.

Coeliac disease

This condition is significantly under-diagnosed; it is believed that at least one in 300 people in the UK suffer from coeliac disease. The exact cause of coeliac disease is unknown. Coeliac disease develops in children (and adults) who are genetically predisposed to the condition, and occurs when eating grains containing gluten. Some children do not develop the disease until a trigger, such as a viral illness or in some cases immunization, begins the abnormal immune response.

Coeliac disease causes the intestine to lose its ability to absorb nutrients. Weight loss, anaemia, and vitamin deficiencies may occur as a result of inadequate absorption of nutrients from the intestinal tract. After exposure to gluten, intestinal damage can develop within a few months but may not become evident for several years. Classic symptoms in adults include abdominal bloating, weight loss, diarrhoea and weakness; presenting factors include fatigue, muscle pain, anaemia, bone and joint pain, infertility and IBS. In children, it's slightly different: diarrhoea, vomiting and abdominal pain are classic symptoms, while constipation/diarrhoea , poor weight gain and food refusal during weaning are common presenting factors.

Because the exact cause is unknown, there is no known way to prevent the development of coeliac disease. However, awareness of risk factors (such as a family member with the disorder) may increase the chance of early diagnosis and treatment. We do know that those at special risk of developing the condition include people with type I diabetes, autoimmune thyroid disease, osteoporosis, dermatitis herpetiformis, epilepsy and Down's syndrome.

Total withdrawal of gluten from the diet permits the intestinal mucosa to heal and results in a disappearance of the symptoms of coeliac disease. Initially, irritability goes away and appetite improves, usually within a matter of days following withdrawal of dietary gluten. A number of studies emphasize the importance of early dietary management to prevent against complications, which can include osteoporosis, cancers, anaemia and infertility.

Becoming gluten-free requires removing all gluten from the diet *for life*. This means eliminating all products that might contain wheat and other offending grains such as rye, oats and barley. Some who are gluten intolerant must even stay away from the presence of gluten. Even if the gluten is not ingested, it can still cause problems. It is important to carefully read all product labels because products labelled wheat-free are not necessarily gluten-free.

Wheat intolerance or allergy?

Recent studies have shown that wheat-intolerant children may actually be allergic or sensitive to the pesticide residues in wheat. Wheat is one of the most heavily sprayed crops in the world, and because the grain is so small, large quantities of pesticides can be absorbed. Some families have found that switching to organic wheat products makes all the difference, and allergies and sensitivities disappear.

Watch out for these terms. Each one of these foods is a type of wheat, or contains wheat:
- durum flour
- couscous
- semolina
- bread crumbs
- kamut
- bulgur
- spelt
- bran
- cereal extract
- enriched flour
- gluten
- high-gluten flour, high-protein flour
- semolina wheat
- wheat bran, wheat germ, wheat gluten, wheat malt, wheat starch
- wholewheat flour

Wheat-intolerant or -allergic children may find it difficult to negotiate a normal diet, as so many 'kid-friendly' foods contain wheat or other grains. Popular breakfast cereals, ordinary bread, cereal bars, biscuits, cakes and many other staples are off the menu, but there are an increasing number of foods now available on the market, which use rice, corn or soya products in place of wheat and wheat products.

Allergic reactions to wheat (IgE-antibody mediated) usually begin within minutes or a few hours after eating or inhaling wheat. The more common symptoms involve the skin, and include urticaria, atopic eczema and facial swelling; the gastrointestinal tract, including abdominal cramps, nausea and vomiting; and the respiratory tract, including asthma or allergic rhinitis.

Wheat and nutrition

Grains are an extremely good source of many vital nutrients, including B vitamins, vitamin E, zinc, magnesium and healthy protein, and these must be replaced in the diet in order to ensure a good healthy balance.

Vegetables contain good levels of the B-complex vitamins, as does wholegrain rice, fish, eggs, dairy produce, yeast, molasses and seeds. The problem is, of course, that many highly allergic people (in particular children) are sensitive to eggs and dairy produce, which can limit intake substantially. The best option is to take a good multi-vitamin and mineral tablet containing the B-complex vitamins, and ensure that a variety of different vegetables are eaten on a daily basis. Marmite is high in B vitamins, as are many pulses (although these can also present problems), and whole rice should be eaten several times a day.

Magnesium is another key nutrient, and because it is implicated in many cases of false food allergy it may be that supplementation – as well as ensuring good dietary levels – can help to rectify multiple food sensitivities. Good natural sources include figs, lemons, grapefruit, sweet corn, almonds, nuts, seeds, dark-green vegetables and apples.

Zinc is found in lamb, beef, pork, yeast, pumpkin seeds, eggs, non-fat dry milk, and nuts, and is essential for immunity.

The following products may contain gluten:
- starch
- dextrin
- malt
- maltodextrin
- HVP (hydrolyzed vegetable protein) fillers
- natural flavourings
- gelatinized starch, edible starch
- modified food starch, modified starch
- soya sauce
- vegetable gum, vegetable starch

Chewing gum may also contain gluten. It is often dusted with wheat flour to prevent stickiness.

Peanuts

Peanut allergies are on the increase, and are a source of great concern for manufacturers and consumers alike. The simple reason is that peanuts can be deadly to a small percentage of the population, and accidental contact or even inhalation of peanut particles, or touching peanut oil, can cause a severe allergic reaction that can lead to anaphylaxis (see page 101).

watch out!

Nowadays labels should be clear if there are peanuts or other nuts contained within a product; in fact, manufacturers must now advise consumers if a product is manufactured in an environment where nuts are also used, even if they are not involved in the processing of the product being labelled. But look out for terms such as:
- peanut extract
- ground nuts
- mixed nuts
- natural flavouring
- arachis oil (which is, in fact, peanut oil)
- ground nut oil

Experts claim that between one and five per cent of the population suffers from a peanut allergy, although this figure is believed to be higher (up to seven per cent) in children.

The peanut is a member of the legume (pulse) family and grown in the ground. It is not considered to be a true nut, although it is regularly referred to as being a 'ground nut'. A peanut allergy is one of the most common food allergies because the peanut proteins can act as powerful allergens, even in tiny quantities, and with minimal contact.

Children under the age of three are most likely to have food sensitivities, probably because their immune systems cannot yet tolerate a wide range of new substances. Children with a family history of food allergies should not be given peanuts or peanut products until at least three, and preferably later, for this reason. Breastfeeding mothers should eliminate peanut products from their own diets. There is also some evidence that avoiding peanuts in the last trimester of pregnancy may also prevent peanut allergy in susceptible children (see pages 178-80).Peanut allergies have doubled in the last five years, according to recent research from the USA. The cause for this is unknown, but the use of soya formulas, the prevalence of peanut oils in skin products, and even vitamins, and children eating peanuts when their immune systems are not mature, are believed to be part of the problem.

Although once considered to be a life-long allergy, recent studies indicate that up to 20 per cent of children diagnosed with peanut allergy outgrow it. For the others, the allergy will be life-long. Adults who develop a peanut allergy are unlikely to outgrow it.

Avoidance is the main way to manage a peanut allergy, and you must be scrupulous to ensure that you do not come into contact with anything that has even minute traces of peanuts, peanut butter or peanut oil. The oil from peanuts tends to linger, so it's also important that cooking, serving and even play equipment does not contain traces. Exposure to peanuts can occur through ingestion, touch or inhalation, and even tiny amounts can trigger a serious reaction.

The peanut allergen is present in both raw and roasted peanuts since it is heat-stable. Peanut oils also contain the peanut allergen, although refined oils may be less problematic for some sufferers.

Foods containing peanuts

A large number of foods, particularly those that are commercially prepared, contain peanuts or peanut products. They are commonly found in:
- processed foods (baked goods and ready meals, for example)
- sweets and chocolate bars
- marzipan
- health bars
- health breads
- mixed nuts
- pastry
- peanut butter
- vegetable oils and fats
- cereals
- biscuits
- dips
- egg rolls
- chocolate
- curry sauces
- some brands of Worcestershire sauce
- ice-cream
- pasta sauces
- African, Chinese, Indonesian, Mexican, Thai, Malaysian and Vietnamese dishes

Many vitamin supplements contain nut oils. Read all labels carefully.

Being careful

Other nuts and nut butters may be fine for peanut allergy sufferers, but most experts recommend avoiding all tree nuts if there is a nut allergy, if only because they are processed, packaged or produced on equipment used for peanuts. One of the nuts that appears to be safest is almonds. Choose organic almonds, wherever possible.

watch out!

It is vitally important that all peanut allergic patients have an action plan in place to deal quickly with an accidental ingestion of peanuts. Most doctors recommend giving an epinephrine (adrenaline) 'EpiPen' (see page 102), which should be carried and used in an emergency. Unlike many food allergies, a peanut allergy is genuinely life threatening, and responsible for many deaths. If you suspect a peanut allergy, see a doctor for advice. Most multiple-allergy sufferers will be checked for peanut allergy as a matter of course, and if it is diagnosed, you must be scrupulous to follow instructions on care and avoidance.

It is important to remember, however, that peanuts are not true nuts, and anyone with a severe peanut allergy must be aware of the relationship between peanuts and other legumes (pulses) such as green peas, chick peas, string beans and soya beans (see page 36). Legumes are often included as ingredients in foods such as hamburgers, baked goods, processed foods and even margarines. Most peanut allergy sufferers are not, however, allergic to other legumes.

If you have a child who is allergic to peanuts, be sure that everyone who feeds and cares for the child knows about the allergy and what to do in case of an attack. Parents should teach allergic children to ask about food they are offered. Most experts believe that banning peanuts at school is not advisable, as it promotes a false sense of security and teaches children nothing about dealing with allergies in the real world. Although there is always risk of contamination, from playground equipment, or in the dining hall, there will, too, be risks throughout their lives and children need to learn to cope.

The most common symptom of peanut allergy is the sudden onset of urticaria (hives) following

Outgrowing the allergy

Children who outgrow peanut allergy have a slight chance of recurrence. This is highly unusual, as there is no other food allergen that has been outgrown and then grown back into. A study from Mount Sinai Hospital's allergy unit in New York reported three children in whom peanut allergies disappeared and then returned later. All three were boys who first developed peanut allergies between a year and 18 months of age. Their peanut allergies disappeared, but then returned when the boys were between six and ten years of age.

But researchers from the Johns Hopkins Children's Center in the USA report that the risk is much lower in children who frequently eat peanuts or peanut products. In a study published in the Journal of Allergy and Clinical Immunology, the Johns Hopkins team recommends that children who outgrow peanut allergy eat concentrated forms of peanut products, such as peanut butter, shelled peanuts or peanut sweets, at least once a month in order to maintain tolerance. In many cases, children who were once allergic are prescribed a teaspoon of peanut butter a day to maintain the results.

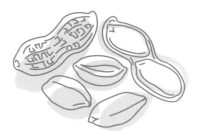

exposure. Itching or swelling of the lips, tongue or mouth are also common early symptoms. Some people may develop swelling of the face, spasm of the bronchial tube and even anaphylaxis (see page 101) following exposure. Some people are so sensitive that they will develop symptoms if they so much as kiss someone who has eaten peanuts or eat out of a dish that has been in contact with peanuts.

Tree nuts

Like peanut allergies, tree nut allergies are common, and potentially life threatening, and they are often life long. Tree nuts may belong to different food families which are unrelated to each other and tree nuts are not related to peanuts (see page 42).

(see page 42)

must know

Types of nut

Tree nuts include:
- almonds
- brazil nuts
- cashews
- chestnuts
- hazelnuts
- hickory nuts
- macadamia nuts
- pecans
- pistachios
- walnuts

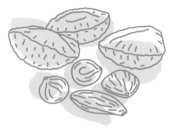

Peanut-allergic people can often eat tree nuts and tree nut-allergic people can often eat peanuts. However, some allergic individuals may be allergic to both peanut and tree nuts. In addition, you can be allergic to some but not all tree nuts.

Nuts may be found as a hidden, unlabelled part of a food because of accidental cross-contamination during manufacturing. Allergic reactions are often caused by eating unlabelled foods, by not checking food labels properly for presence of nuts, or from foods which contain hidden unlabelled nuts.

It is also important to avoid any product labelled 'may contain nuts'. Manufacturers use this term if they cannot guarantee that a food they are producing is free of nuts, usually because nuts are being used in the same machines for other foods. A company that makes similar foods with and without nuts may have difficulty cleaning the machines in between processing the different foods, or packages may be mislabelled. Because machines are typically cleaned with water, which does not remove traces of oils, it is quite likely that when a food containing nuts is put through the machine, traces of nuts remain on the machine. The first batches of foods made without nuts to go through the same machine will likely contain traces of nuts. These foods must be avoided.

Some sufferers are only allergic to one family of nuts and so other nuts are safe to eat. The nuts within each family share certain characteristics, which makes them more likely to affect susceptible people with allergies to another nut in the same family. However, trying nuts from other families should only be undertaken very cautiously, and preferably in the safety of a hospital. Skin prick and RAST tests (see pages 77-79) should be able to identify specific nut allergies, so if the results of these prove negative, you may be safe to try nuts from different nut families. The families are: Walnut (walnut and pecan); Birch (hazelnut and hickory nuts); Mango (pistachio and cashews); Plum (almond); Legythis (brazil); Macadamia and Beech (beechnut and chestnut). Similarly, foods such as water chestnut, pine nut (pignolia or pinyon nuts), coconut, or nutmeg do not need to be avoided by nut-allergic people unless they are also allergic to these foods. These allergies are rare.

Like most true food allergies, an allergic reaction to tree nuts usually begins within minutes, but may be delayed for up to four hours. Symptoms, which include burning or tingling on the lips, tongue or mouth, hives, blotching on the face, an immediate runny nose, sneezing and itching, watery eyes, coughing, vomiting, cramps, choking, wheezing, trouble breathing and diarrhoea, can last for up to a day. The allergic reaction can stop at any stage, or may progress to anaphylaxis (see page 101).

Anyone with severe nut allergy should avoid tree nuts completely, and read labels carefully to avoid accidental intake. Anyone with severe nut allergy should have and be able to use an EpiPen (see page 102) as soon as they begin to react to the accidental ingestion of these nuts.

The following products may contain nuts, and care should be taken to read the labels:
- chocolate
- sweets
- puddings and desserts
- almond paste (marzipan)
- doughnuts
- breakfast cereals
- muesli bars
- pesto
- chocolate bars
- sunscreens
- shampoos
- bath oils
- popcorns
- speciality cheese spreads
- some coffees
- muffins, biscuits and other baked goods
- Crosse & Blackwell Worcestershire sauce
- chocolate nut spreads
- some liqueurs
- hotdog and hamburger buns
- flavoured crisps
- nut butters
- ice-creams
- Chinese, Thai, Indian and Indonesian dishes
- ready-prepared sandwiches
- breads
- almond mocha
- almond extract

Sesame seeds

Sesame seeds are becoming increasingly popular in Western diets, and are also one of the key allergens known to cause food allergies. They are extremely potent allergens and can cause severe allergic reactions (anaphylaxis) in susceptible individuals.

watch out!

Because of their size, sesame seeds often cross-contaminate other products; for example, they easily fall off burger buns in fast-food restaurants, and make their way into foods that you may assume are safe. Avoid consuming food from any restaurant or take-away where sesame seeds are used.

Sesame is used extensively in the food industry and the seeds present a danger because of their versatility. They have been identified in non-sesame products, especially bread, due to cross-contamination. Sesame is also known as Benne, Gingelly, Til or Teel, Simsin and Anjonjoli on foreign products.

Interestingly, awareness of sesame allergy is low. It is less common than peanut allergy, but allergic reactions can be just as severe. One of the greatest difficulties facing sufferers is the fact that it is hidden in so many foods.

In a recent report, doctors monitored published reports of allergic reactions to sesame products from 1950 (the first documented case of an allergic reaction to sesame) to the present. They noted that a study of Australian children showed that allergic reactions to sesame ranked fourth behind reactions to egg, milk and peanuts, and sesame was the third most common allergy-inducing food in Israeli children.

Some people may have tree nut and peanut allergies in addition to a sesame allergy, while others will not. You will need to be tested (see pages 77-79) in order to determine the exact nature of your allergy if you haven't already had a reaction after ingesting the sesame seeds. It is worth noting, too, that a sesame seed allergy does not necessarily mean an allergy to all seeds. In fact, many sufferers are able to eat most other seeds (sunflower being an exception, as it is from the same family as sesame seeds) without a problem. It is also possible to be allergic to sesame seeds and not sunflower seeds. Individual testing is required.

Reaction to sesame is much the same as that of tree nuts and peanuts, and the same care should be exercised. Parents of sufferers and sufferers should be aware of how to react quickly to accidental ingestion. Like most true food allergies, however, complete avoidance of sesame is necessary. This is not always easy, particularly when eating out, but it must be undertaken. Avoid all products that say 'may contain traces of sesame', as this is a fallback for manufacturers who cannot confirm whether sesame is present or not.

Interestingly, however, a 2005 study found that 91 per cent of severe reactions occurred when sesame seeds or sesame oil were used deliberately as an ingredient rather than as an accidental ingredient. But 65 per cent of reactions occurred on the first exposure to sesame seeds, and 94 per cent of those who tested positive to sesame seed allergy were also allergic to tree nuts or peanuts. The simple solution is to get an allergy test if you suspect that sesame seeds cause you to suffer a reaction.

Foods containing sesame include:
- hummus
- tahini
- halvah
- baked goods
- biscuits
- chocolate bars
- muesli bars
- health foods
- dips
- sauces (particularly Chinese and other oriental foods such as Japanese, Indonesian and Thai)
- sausages
- processed meats
- vegetarian burgers
- chutneys
- stir-fries
- risottos
- patés
- marinades
- salads
- bagels
- sesame oils (all forms)
- spice mixtures
- pretzels
- sesame salt
- tempeh
- herbal drinks (such as Aqua Libra)
- pharmaceutical products, such as plasters, liniments, ointments and soaps
- cosmetics, where it may be listed as sesamum indicum

Fish

Fish allergies have become increasingly common over the past decade, and unlike many other allergies, they are not normally outgrown. In fact, in many sufferers, the symptoms become worse with repeated exposure to fish.

must know

Fish allergies
Fish are roughly grouped into five families; allergy to one 'family' or species does not necessarily mean allergy to others, but ask for your doctor or specialist to test out your susceptibility rather than trying new fish yourself. The groupings families are:
Chordate Laminiformes: shark
Salmoniformes: salmon, trout, pike
Gadiformes: cod, haddock, hake
Perciformes: snapper, mackerel, tuna, bonito, grouper
Pleurenectiformes: sole, flounder, halibut, plaice

The protein in the flesh of fish is what most commonly causes the allergic reaction. However, it is also possible to have an allergic reaction to fish gelatine, made from the skin and bones of fish. Although fish oil does not contain protein from the fish from which it was extracted, it is likely to be contaminated with small molecules of protein and therefore should be avoided.

If you are allergic to one species of fish, such as cod, you will often react to other types of fish, such as hake, haddock, mackerel and whiting, which are part of the same 'family'. The allergens in each species or 'family' of fish are quite similar. Some sufferers are only allergic to a specific species, and can tolerate other types of fish. Salmon and cod, for example, are from different 'families' of fish. However, experts do not recommend that you experiment if you suffer from any type of fish allergy. Ask for a test to assess your risk. Fish allergies can be very dangerous.

Cooking does not alter the allergens in fish; in fact, there is some evidence that people who are allergic to fish can tolerate raw fish (such as that used in sushi), but not cooked fish.

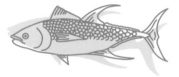

Not always an allergy

When fish is not chilled correctly, or begins to spoil, histamine (the same chemical that our bodies produce when we suffer from an allergy) is produced. This causes symptoms that are very similar to allergic reactions, when it is, in fact, a type of food poisoning (histamine fish poisoning, or HFP). Tuna, mackerel, sardines and mahi-mahi are most commonly implicated in incidents of histamine poisoning. The fish are non-toxic when caught, but increase in histamine content as bacterial numbers increase. They may look and smell normal, and cooking does not destroy the histamine. So what appears to be a fish allergy, may well be poisoning.

The symptoms include nausea, vomiting, diarrhoea, an oral burning sensation or peppery taste, hives, itching, red rash, and high blood pressure. The onset of the symptoms usually occurs within a few minutes after ingestion of the implicated food and the duration of symptom ranges from a few hours to 24 hours. Antihistamines can be used effectively to treat this type of poisoning.

Furthermore, allergic reactions to a parasitic worm, *Anisakis*, that is often found in various fish species, has been described in people eating fish, and can mimic a fish sensitivity. This worm is a common intestinal parasite found in fish and other seafood. It is considered to be a food allergen and to induce IgE-mediated reactions. Hypersensitivity to Anisakis is an unusual cause of anaphylaxis but it should always be borne in mind in countries where a great deal of fish is consumed, especially if it is eaten raw or undercooked.

watch out!

Some ingredients are derived from fish, and may not be immediately obvious. Look out for:
- omega-3 supplements
- chilli
- any food containing gelatine (check source)
- roe
- caviar
- surimi (imitation crab made from white fish)
- agar
- alginic Acid
- alginate
- anchovies
- disodium ionsinate

Fish or shellfish

Generally speaking, allergy to fish does not suggest a similar allergy to shellfish, but in some people both allergies occur. For safety reasons, a fish allergy usually precludes eating any type of fish, just as an allergy to one type of shellfish means that all should be avoided. Fish allergies are more common in children, whereas shellfish allergies tend to affect more adults.

Interestingly, in countries (such as those in Scandinavia) where fish is eaten frequently, fish allergies are highest. In Sweden, for example, some 39 per cent of children are allergic to fish. The reason for the rise is unclear, but it may be linked to the fact that more and more fish is farmed, fish products are used increasingly in processed foods, and the processing of fish itself has changed quite dramatically over the past few years, with milk solutions being used instead of water, thereby adding in more potential allergens. There is also some evidence that breastfed babies can be sensitized to cod through their mothers' milk. In general, about 22 per cent of the population is allergic or sensitive to fish.

If you suffer from a fish allergy, strictly avoiding fish and food containing fish products is the only way to prevent a reaction. For some individuals, canned tuna appears to be acceptable, but check with your allergy specialist before trying it. Children with a strong history of allergies in the family (food allergies and atopic conditions, for example) should avoid fish and seafood for the first two or three years of life, and begin with canned tuna (which is the least allergenic form of fish). Otherwise, fish can normally be introduced at about 12 months.

Fish-allergic individuals should avoid fish and seafood restaurants because of the risk of contamination. Moreover, fish protein can become airborne during cooking and cause an allergic reaction. Some highly allergic people will suffer a reaction simply by walking through a fish market, or standing near a fish counter. It is important to remember that allergic reactions to fish can be severe, and are often a cause of anaphylaxis (see page 101). All sufferers should be taught how to administer adrenaline (in the form of an EpiPen), and carry it with them at all times (see page 102).

Common reactions include skin, stomach, or respiratory problems. More specifically they can include nasal congestion, hives, itching, swelling, wheezing or shortness of breath, nausea, upset stomach, cramps, heart burn, wind, diarrhoea, light-headedness, or fainting. Reactions usually appear within two hours of ingestion, inhaling cooking vapours, or handling of seafood. However, it has been reported the reactions can be delayed as long as 24 hours.

Getting the right nutrients

Fish and shellfish are an excellent source of protein. Oily fish, in particular, is a rich source of vitamin A, vitamin D, omega-3 fatty acids (an essential fatty acid or EFA, which is required for learning, growth and development, and also linked to immunity and preventing allergies) and calcium.

It is the EFAs found in fish that are most important for health, but these can be replaced by drizzling flaxseed oil over meals, and adding plenty of fresh seeds to the menu. Selenium is an important mineral, but it is found in good quantities in onions, tomatoes, broccoli and wheatgerm (providing you are not wheat or gluten intolerant).

Look for calcium in leafy green vege-tables, fortified foods and drinks, and dairy produce to replace the calcium you are lacking from eating oily fish (see page 31).

watch out!

Food labels need to be read carefully because highly processed foods may contain hidden fish or shellfish. For example, the basis for imitation crab, lobster and prawns is pollock. It can also be used in beef and pork substitutes as part of hot dogs, ham, and pizza toppings. Fish skin is used to clarify some coffees and wines, and other parts of fish are used in Worcestershire sauce, many Asian meals, Caesar salad, salad dressings, cooking sauces, condiments and much, much more.

By law, fish or fish products must be noted on the label of all foods, but this ruling was only made in 2005, and products may predate it. Look, too, at the list of foods on page 55, as the distinction between fish and shellfish is often blurred, and may both fall under the umbrella term 'seafood'.

Shellfish

Shellfish allergies are even more common than fish allergies, and are also known as 'seafood' allergies. However, as we mentioned earlier, a shellfish allergy does not necessarily mean that you will also suffer from an allergy to fish.

must know
Preservatives
Shellfish are often treated with preservatives known as benzoates after they are caught. In some cases, suspected allergy to shellfish is, in fact, a reaction to these chemicals.

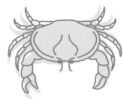

To complicate things further, 'shellfish' traditionally includes abalone, clam, cockle (periwinkle, sea urchin), conch, limpets, mussels, octopus, oysters, periwinkle, quahaugs, scallops, snails (escargot), squid (calamari) and whelks. This group is known as 'molluscs', while another name – 'crustaceans' – is given to crab, crayfish (crawfish, écrevisse), lobster (langouste, langoustine, coral, tomalley), prawns and shrimp (crevette). Both crustaceans and molluscs cause a shellfish allergy and must be avoided.

Prawns appear to be the worst offender, causing respiratory problems in most sufferers, and crab is also a powerful allergen to many people. A higher prevalence of shellfish allergy is found in the countries where it is a staple part of the diet, such as Scandinavian countries, Spain and Japan.

Shellfish contains potent allergens, which affect sensitized individuals and cause life-threatening adverse reactions that are usually life long. Extreme sensitivity to minute quantities of shellfish is occasionally noted, and even exposure to cooking fumes is enough to cause reactions in certain individuals. Sufferers are often aware of traces of shellfish in foods, because they experience a burning of the mouth, lips and tongue, often with the first bite.

Like those who suffer from fish allergies, it is recommended that shellfish allergy sufferers avoid restaurants where shellfish is a main part of the menu, and should always ask whether any shellfish was used in the preparation of other foods.

Possible sources of fish, crustaceans and shellfish

As mentioned earlier, the line between shellfish and fish is often blurred, and the term 'seafood' may be used to include either or both. It's worth checking the label carefully to ensure that your particular allergens are not included. Remember, too, that foods purchased on the internet or in international shops may not be subject to the same rigorous labelling system, so care should be taken.

- coffee
- cold meats (such as ham and salami)
- dips, spreads, kamaboko (imitation crab/lobster meat)
- ethnic foods, such as paella, spring rolls, fried rice
- fish mixtures, such as surimi (used to make imitation crab/lobster meat)
- garnishes, such as antipasti, caponata (Sicilian relish), caviar, roe (unfertilized fish eggs)
- gelatine
- marshmallows
- hot dogs
- pizza toppings
- salad dressings
- sauces, such as fish, marinara, steak, Worcestershire
- soups
- ready-prepared sandwiches
- spreads, such as taramasalata (contains salted carp roe)
- sushi
- wine

Non-food sources of fish and shellfish:
- fish food
- pet food
- some food supplements, such as glucosamine

Reactions usually occur within two hours of ingestion or handling of shellfish, or even inhaling cooking vapours. Reactions can also be delayed for up to six hours, as has been frequently reported for species such as abalone and squid. The more common symptoms include skin, stomach and respiratory problems, similar to those experienced with fish (see page 51).

Other foods

The difficult aspect of food allergies is that many sufferers have multiple allergies, and not just to the main eight culprits. Similarly, some sufferers have no reaction to the 'big eight', and have other allergies that are more difficult to pinpoint.

did you know?

Studies show that 175 foods, outside the 'big eight', have been shown to produce allergic reactions in susceptible people. In many cases, allergies to specific foods are geographical – celery allergy is common in some European countries, sesame seeds in the Middle East (due to the popularity of tahini), and buckwheat in southeast Asia.

Theoretically, any susceptible person can develop an allergy to any food. Symptoms can be dramatic, or they can be fairly innocuous, which makes detection even harder. Moreover, many of the other common food allergens are 'ingredients' in other dishes and food products, so pinpointing them can be difficult. Some of the most common foods to affect susceptible people are corn (maize), yeast, citrus fruit (which includes tomatoes, oranges, grapefruit, lemons, etc.), coffee, chocolate, sulphites and mustard.

Corn (maize)

Just as fish allergies are common in countries who consume large quantities of fish, so corn allergies are also more prevalent in countries such as the US, largely because it is present in so many prepared foods (in the form of corn flour, cornmeal and corn syrup, for example). Although these products are used in the UK and Europe, they are not used to the same degree. Corn is implicated in many cases of food intolerance, and is less likely to cause true allergies.

It is often difficult to pinpoint a corn allergy, largely because it is almost impossible to eliminate every source of corn from your diet. Symptoms from corn allergy can, however, be as severe as other food allergens, so it is important that sufferers make a concerted effort to keep their diet as low in corn and corn products as possible.

The element of corn that causes symptoms is the corn protein, not the oil. During the processing of corn oil, the protein is removed, therefore making it safe for most people suffering from corn allergy.

Like all allergies, symptoms can differ greatly among sufferers. Traditional symptoms of corn allergy include: asthma attacks, shortness of breath, breathing difficulties, difficulty swallowing, tingling in mouth, tongue and lips, stomach cramps, discomfort and pain, nausea and/or vomiting, diarrhoea, migraines, rashes and hives. Anaphylaxis (see page 101) may also result. Other sufferers report depression, eczema, fatigue, joint pains, recurring ear infections, respiratory problems and disturbed sleep, although these symptoms are considered 'non-traditional'.

Because of the potential severity of the condition, and because so many medications and even some intravenous (IV) solutions can contain corn derivatives, experts recommend that sufferers wear a medic alert bracelet, as well as carrying emergency medication, such as an EpiPen (see page 102).

Other products that may contain corn

Corn oil may be used in emollients, toothpastes, cosmetics, adhesives for envelopes, stamps and stickers. Cling film, paper cups and paper plates may also be coated with corn oil. Check the label of medication, too. Hidden sources of corn include throat lozenges, ointments, suppositories, vitamins, laxatives, capsules, liquid medication and aspirin.

watch out!
Other foods associated with severe allergic reactions include poppy seeds, sunflower seeds, peas, lentils and chickpeas. In many cases, severe reactions occur after large amounts have been eaten, rather than accidental contamination; in some cases, allergies suddenly crop up after years of successfully eating a food.

Foods that contain corn

Some corn products are fairly obvious, and are, therefore, very easy to eliminate from the diet. Tortillas, tortilla chips, cornflakes, sweetcorn and popcorn are obvious targets. But, remember that many processed foods are made with corn syrup, corn flour or cornmeal.

Avoid eating products that contain:
- whole corn
- corn flour
- corn starch
- cereal starch
- edible starch
- custard powder
- corn on the cob
- sweetcorn
- polenta
- corn alcohol
- corn gluten
- corn sugar
- corn syrup
- corn sweetener
- corn meal
- corn oil
- popcorn

The following ingredients may also be based on corn:
- dextrose (also known as glucose or corn sugar)
- dextrin
- dextrates
- maltodextrin
- caramel
- malt syrup

Look out for corn or its derivatives in:

- pasta sauces
- some baked beans
- tinned soups/soup mixes
- ready meals and sauces
- cornbread
- some peanut butters
- processed meats
- imitation seafood
- imitation corn
- low-allergen products designed to replace wheat
- baked goods
- ice-cream
- sports drinks
- chips
- fish fingers
- crisps
- sauces
- salad dressings
- caramel flavouring
- biscuits
- sweets
- some soft drinks and even fruit drinks
- maple and nut flavouring
- corn starch (added to most icing sugar and baking powders to keep them from caking or clumping)
- marshmallows
- vegetable gums and starches (not all; check with manufacturers)
- some food starches and modified food starches
- some may be contained in distilled white vinegar, bleached white flour and iodized table salt

Foods with yeast

- all breads and anything that uses yeast to help it rise
- foods covered in breadcrumbs
- Twiglets
- pizzas
- bread pudding
- alcohol
- citrus fruit drinks and juices
- malted milk, malted drinks
- malted cereals
- cereals enriched with vitamins
- some salad dressings
- some mayonnaise
- a variety of condiments (such as mustard, vinegar, Worcestershire sauce, horseradish sauce, ketchup, barbeque sauces
- hamburgers, sausages and cooked meats made with bread or breadcrumbs
- yeast extracts (Bisto, Marmite, Oxo, Bovril, Vegemite, gravy browning, etc.)
- all B-vitamin preparations, unless otherwise stated
- any food that has been fermented for a long time

Yeast

A fairly new allergy to be recognized is yeast, which presents itself as both intolerance and true allergy. Some sufferers experience immediate, full-blown, painful and debilitating symptoms upon eating yeast or products that contain it, while in others symptoms are more insidious, causing pain, fatigue, general achiness, poor sleep, digestive problems, and persistent rhinitis (runny nose). The prevalence of yeast allergies is largely unknown, but it is believed to be related to the condition candida (see page 172), in which the yeast candida albicans overgrows in the body. Candida is still a widely disputed condition, but yeast allergy is undoubtedly accepted, and appears to affect a small percentage of the population.

A true allergy to yeast means avoiding all foods that contain it; even those who are intolerant, and can stomach small quantities, are advised to go as 'yeast-free' as possible.

Sulphites

Another problem is sulphites, which are sometimes used to preserve the colour of foods such as dried fruits and vegetables, and to inhibit the growth of micro-organisms in fermented foods such as wine. Sulphites are also often sprayed on fruits and vegetables, and used in a variety of ready-made and processed foods. Some ingredients, such as bleached (white) flour, have been treated with sulphites in the early stages of manufacturing, and may not, therefore, be listed as an 'ingredient' or additive on the label.

Sulphites are safe for most people. A small segment of the population, however, has been found to develop shortness of breath or fatal shock shortly after exposure to these preservatives. The reason is that sulphites give off a gas called sulphur dioxide, that can irritate the airways of asthmatics. Therefore sulphites are capable of producing severe asthma attacks in sulphite-sensitive asthmatics – in fact, it is estimated to occur in five to 20 per cent of asthmatics, particularly those with severe asthma, or in those whose asthma is poorly controlled. Reactions can be mild through to life threatening.

Occasionally sufferers exposed to sulphites will experienced symptoms similar to anaphylaxis, with flushing, fast heartbeat, wheezing, hives, dizziness, stomach upset and diarrhoea, collapse, tingling or difficulty swallowing. Other sufferers experience symptoms affecting the skin, such as rashes, itchiness and hives.

Sulphites

These can often be found in the following foods:
- anything treated with sulphur dioxide
- lemon, lime and grape juice
- ready-prepared salads
- fresh fruit and vegetables
- wines and beer
- ready-prepared sandwiches
- cordials and some fruit juices
- some soft drinks
- vinegar
- dry potatoes
- some gravies and sauces
- fruit toppings and maraschino cherries
- pickled onions
- maple syrup
- jellies and gelatine
- bread, pie or pizza dough
- dried fruits
- some crustaceans (sulphur is often added on top to stop discolouring)
- some sausages
- coconut
- many topical and injectible medications, including adrenaline, some eye drops, some corticosteroids.

Ask your pharmacist for details

must know

Sulphur dioxide
The following preservatives give off sulphur dioxide (which can cause asthma attacks in some susceptible people): sodium sulphite, sodium hydrogen sulphite, sodium metabisulphite, potassium metabisulphite, and calcium sulphite.
Packaged food often contains sulphites and metabisulphites, but these are easier to avoid as they are declared on the label as E numbers E220-E227.

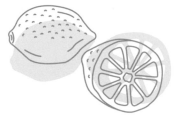

Citrus fruits

Citrus fruits, such as oranges, clementines, tangerines, grapefruit, lemons and limes have been known to cause allergies in a small number of people, and some of these have been considered life threatening (see anaphylaxis, page 101). In some cases, the seed proteins may be responsible for causing allergic reactions such as urticaria (hives), asthma or eczema. In some cases, the peel and oils from the fruit appear to be the main culprits, in particular causing skin problems such as rashes and dermatitis, rather than the juice itself. Citrus fruits also contain many aromatic substances, colours and a chemical called tyramine, which might cause hypersensitivity and reactions that are not true allergies. Similarly, citrus fruits contain high concentrations of chlorogenic acid that may be responsible for many of the symptoms thought to be allergic. An allergy test will need to be undertaken to confirm a true allergy.

Coffee

An allergy to coffee is also fairly new in terms of being diagnosed and/or even suspected; however, the increase in coffee bars, flavoured coffees and coffee-containing drinks has sparked a spate of allergy, and many sufferers are unaware that coffee is the culprit. Once again, it is difficult to know which element of coffee is the problem. Some sufferers are allergic to the caffeine in coffee, which means that they also experience reactions to chocolate, tea and caffeine-containing soft drinks.

Others are allergic to coffee itself. Still others are allergic or sensitive to the variety of different chemicals used in the production and manufacture of coffee and coffee-containing products. Coffee (particularly instant) can contain up to 300 different chemical agents, any of which can spark a reaction in sensitive individuals. It's a heavily sprayed crop, too, which means that fertilizers and pesticides may be to blame for some symptoms.

Symptoms can be dramatic in some individuals, particularly those allergic to the caffeine, and can even lead to delirium, trembling, restlessness and severe anxiety. Caffeine is a drug, and studies show that the longer people are exposed to this drug, the higher the chances of developing an intolerance and an allergy. Once this happens, caffeine-allergic people can not properly metabolize caffeine, which then goes on to literally 'poison' the body and brain. The problem, too, is that caffeine is stimulating, which tends to mask its allergic symptoms. When people drink coffee, adrenaline increases. Of course, the emergency treatment of choice for severe (life threatening) allergic reactions is adrenaline, which can make things much worse for caffeine-allergy sufferers.

Symptoms of coffee allergy include skin problems (eczema in particular appears to flare up), rashes, hives, itchy skin, stomach cramps, diarrhoea and/or nausea, headaches and migraine, fatigue and, in rare cases, anaphylaxis. Many sufferers have an instant reaction, while others simply feel unwell and under the weather, even hours later.

must know

Citrus
Avoid all foods that contain citrus juice, citrus fruit or oils, particularly if you are not sure of the element to which you are allergic. Look out for:
• fruit puddings
• fruit-flavoured sweets
• 'naturally sweetened' foods, which may use fruit juice
• fruit salads
• some salad dressings
• fruit jams and jellies
• fruit baked goods, including fruit pies and tarts
• fruit juices
• some cleaners and air fresheners (many contain orange and lemon oils)
• foods containing 'zest' of any citrus fruit and many, many more

Chocolate

Studies show that true chocolate allergies are fairly rare; in fact, many cases of 'chocolate allergy' are simply allergies to its ingredients, which can include soya, milk, vanilla, flavourings, nuts and caffeine (see pages 76-77). Some people have undoubtedly reacted strongly to chocolate, and suffered unreproducible symptoms, such as rashes, hives, headaches and migraine, digestive discomfort, diarrhoea, vomiting and a general feeling of malaise. There are recorded cases, too, of people reacting dramatically, and suffering a life-threatening reaction. Thankfully, these are very, very rare.

Interestingly, several research studies have found that people who suffer from multiple allergies often have a reaction to a skin prick test (see pages 77-79) when the cocoa bean is tested; however, they do not experience any real symptoms of allergy when eating cocoa or chocolate in any form. The cocoa bean undergoes a dramatic manufacturing process before it becomes chocolate, and there is some evidence to suggest that this process destroys any potential allergens. If you suspect a chocolate allergy, ensure that your specialist tests for chocolate, and not just cocoa. There is a very high chance that you will not be allergic.

Mustard

Mustard allergy is quite rare in the UK, but it is more common in other European countries, such as France and Spain, where it has been reported to cause severe reactions, including anaphylaxis. Larger studies in allergic individuals suggest that mustard allergy may account for one to seven per cent of food

watch out!

Apart from the 'big eight', more than 175 foods have been identified as causing allergy in susceptible people. However, many of these allergies are outgrown, after a period of elimination, although fish, nut, shellfish and tree nut allergies are often lifelong. If you suspect a food allergy, it is very important to have a food allergy test (see page 77). Not all allergies are obvious. Other common foods causing allergic reactions are, for example, strawberries (which contain salicylates), kiwi, pine nuts, celery, peppers, aubergine, tomatoes, coconuts, spices and even rice. In reality, no food is 'safe' and any food has the potential to cause a reaction.

allergies in the regions in which they were carried out. Mustard allergens are heat-resistant and do not break down easily, and therefore are not markedly affected by food processing.

French researchers found that allergic reactions to mustard start very early in life, usually under three years of age. Frequent contact with mustard in infancy could be explained by the presence of mustard in baby foods in glass pots for babies and commercial foods for toddlers. Breastfeeding mothers may also sensitize children through their breast milk. Thankfully, reactions in children do not appear to be as dramatic as those in adults; however, digestive discomfort, hives, flaring of eczema, rhinitis, and breathing difficulties may be experienced in adults and children alike.

People who are allergic to mustard will react to any food that comes from the mustard plant, including jars of mustard, mustard powder, mustard leaves, seeds and flowers, sprouted mustard seeds, mustard oil, and foods that contain these. Mustard is used as an ingredient in many foods, including salad dressings, sauces, marinades, ready-prepared foods (including sandwiches and some soups), salads and some baked goods. Remember that many topical preparations, such as those for arthritis and even chest colds or bronchitis, may contain mustard oil.

Traditional mustard and cress contains seedlings grown from mustard seeds and because it generally isn't pre-packed, it wouldn't have to be labelled as containing mustard. But much of what is sold as 'cress' in the UK comes from other plants and doesn't include any mustard.

want to know more?

If you suffer from lactose intolerance, lactase drops or tablets may allow you to digest small quantities of dairy produce without symptoms. Visit www.lactose.co.uk to purchase, and for details of stockists.

Lactofree is the UK's first virtually lactose-free milk, with only 0.5 per cent lactose. For more information, recipes and stockists, visit their website: www.lactofree.co.uk.

Coeliac sufferers can find invaluable advice, recipes and up-to-date research at The Coeliac Disease Society. Visit www.coeliac.co.uk or ring 01494 437278).

The very best source for online allergy-free foods is www.wheatanddairyfree. com.

The Food Standards Agency has a wealth of information and advice on their website: www.eatwell.gov.uk.

The Flour Advisory Bureau provides information on flour and bread intolerance/ allergies. Visit www.wheatintolerance. co.uk.

Visit Food You Can Eat, for free recipes, divided by allergen: www.foodyoucaneat.com.

Case study

Multiple food allergies

Laura

Both of Laura's parents suffered from eczema and her father had been asthmatic since he was a child, although neither had any experience of food allergies. Having been warned during her pregnancy that two atopic (see page 19) parents would increase the likelihood of their child suffering from allergies, Laura's mother was not surprised that Laura had an instant reaction to formula milk at two weeks of age. She suffered from colic and became very fussy, and soon went on to vomit after every feed. She was switched to a special infant formula, known as a hydrolyzed formula (see page 137) and her growth and development were considered to be fine. Problems started, however, when she began to be weaned, and it soon became clear that a number of foods produced a violent reaction, and others caused her to suffer from rashes, itching, and bouts of eczema. By the age of three it became clear that the worst offenders were nuts, seeds, cow's milk, eggs, and wheat. She also became fussy, irritable and itchy when she was given tomatoes, citrus fruit and tuna, while bananas caused welts to form on her lips. With the advice of a dietitian and an allergy specialist,

Laura was given a bland, allergen-free diet, which consisted mainly of rice, soya and corn products, with plenty of leafy green vegetables and pulses to ensure she was getting adequate nutrition. It became clear, too, that peanuts were a particular worry, and she suffered instant breathing problems if any were accidentally ingested. This meant advising her nursery and then school of the problem, where an immediate 'nut ban' was put into place. She also carried an EpiPen, in the event that she came into contact with peanuts in any form. Other foods were added to the list in infancy, and after a series of allergy tests. However, after three years of a completely allergen-free diet, Laura was soon able to tolerate small amounts of all of the foods to which she had become allergic, including peanuts. On the advice of her specialist, she now has a teaspoon of peanut butter every day to ensure that her symptoms do not return (see page 45). Her diet is full and varied, and although she has mild reactions to some foods, such as milk and tomatoes, when she is run down or ill, she has outgrown her food allergies completely. Laura is now nine, and shows no signs of any significant allergies, and has outgrown her eczema as well.

3 Identification

Diagnosing a food allergy can be complicated and time consuming. First and foremost, it is ultimately very important to recognize that food is causing the symptoms. Many other health conditions share their symptoms with allergies, and eliminating foods without proper diagnosis can affect your overall health and nutritional status. In this chapter we will look at how to pinpoint food allergies, as well as looking at sensible elimination diets and the variety of tests that can be undertaken to confirm the foods to which you may be allergic.

First steps

Many people have become aware over time that different foods make them feel uncomfortable or even ill, and in many instances they simply avoid them – sometimes even unconsciously. It is, however, always worth pinpointing food allergies and those foods to which you may have become intolerant or sensitive.

> **must know**
>
> **Is it an allergy?**
> Not all cases of suspected food allergy are, in fact, true allergies or intolerance. For example, food additives such as colourants and preservatives may trigger pseudo-allergic reactions. These are not IgE mediated, but may cause the release of histamine (see opposite page).

Niggling symptoms in the latter cases may not cause any real threat to quality of life and health; however, removing food from the diet can improve the way you feel immeasurably. In the case of true food allergies, many sufferers experience increasingly serious reactions with every exposure, and this should be addressed. Moreover, many foods are used as ingredients in other products, and during manufacturing processes, and unless you are clear about the foods with which you have a problem, you will never successfully remove them from your diet. Awareness is the most important part of prevention.

It is also important to remember that health problems may not be linked to food. Many other illnesses can mimic the symptoms of food allergy, and it is necessary to establish that food is the cause – or rule it out – so that a proper diagnosis can be made. Some cases of food poisoning (such as in the case of fish, see page 50) have been put down to food allergies, and sufferers are pleasantly surprised to find that foods that they thought were off the menu are actually absolutely fine to eat. Similarly, when we are rundown or ill, taking medication, or following a course of antibiotics, some foods may cause a reaction. Upon returning to full health, or ceasing the medication, symptoms cease.

Similarly, certain foods, particularly fruit and vegetables, can cause reactions such as itching or rashes when they touch the lips and mouth. This is called oral allergy syndrome (see page 100).

These reactions usually occur in people who suffer from hay fever and are sensitive to pollen: for example, pollen from birch, grass, or plants in the daisy family such as ragweed and mugwort. The allergens in these types of pollen are also found in some fruit and vegetables. Someone sensitive to ragweed pollen may suffer an oral reaction when they eat melon. The good news is that cooking often destroys the allergens that cause this kind of reaction to fresh fruit and vegetables, so suffering symptoms may not mean cutting these out of your diet for good.

Interestingly, too, some people suffer from a condition called 'exercise-induced food allergy', which basically means that they suffer a reaction when they take exercise within a couple of hours of eating a particular food. In this case, they may well be able to tolerate specific foods, as long as they avoid exercise after eating.

So, it is clear the food allergies are far from being clear cut, and there may be many other factors causing or exacerbating your reactions. What's more, they may also be short-term or easily avoidable, which makes the need to alter your diet less important. This is one reason why keeping a food diary is so important. And we'll talk about that next.

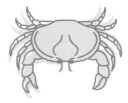

Keeping a diary

In order to work out a food allergy or intolerance, you'll need to keep a food diary of everything that passes your lips – not just meals, but also drinks, food supplements and even water.

Record the time that each is eaten or drunk, the approximate quantities, and relevant details, such as the brand and whether or not the food or drink is organic. Write all of these details on the left-hand page of a large notebook. On the right-hand page record any symptoms that you notice, the time they occur and how long they last. Make a note of any obvious changes in behaviour or mood, any rashes that might appear, or hives, or changes in bowel movements. Vomiting, diarrhoea, tingling of the mouth or lips, breathing difficulties or even wheeziness should also be noted, as, too, should skin changes. An exacerbation of eczema may be an obvious clue.

It is also important to note down anything that may affect your symptoms. If you are a woman, are you menstruating or pre-menstrual? Changes in mood, bowel habits, sleep patterns and overall wellbeing often happen during this period and may have nothing to do with food. Consider, too, any medication you are taking – and check the leaflet accompanying it for any side effects. This may explain some of the symptoms you are experiencing. If you are ill, under stress, rundown, or have just

must know

Elimination diet

An elimination diet is virtually the only fail-safe way to know if you are intolerant (see pages 82-91). There are a number of specialists who work in the field of allergy medicine, including doctors, registered dietitians, nutritionists, consultants, immunologists and, for young children, paediatric specialists. You can be referred to any of these specialists by your GP, or other health professional.

finished a course of antibiotics, your reactions may also be different, and this must be taken into consideration.

At the end of a week or so, go through the diary, looking for recurring patterns. You may notice that you become moody, tired or experience stomach cramps after eating toast or bread, that you have a headache after eating a banana or some sesame seeds, or suffer from itchiness and a rash around your mouth after eating cheese.

Make a comprehensive list of every food that seems to trigger a regular pattern of symptoms. Watch out too for foods that you regularly crave, as these may well be some of the main culprits (see page 85). And think about foods to which you have a natural aversion – eggs, for example, or milk.

If you are slightly confused about what the exact culprits might be, try another week, but keep your diet as simple as possible. For example, if you regularly experience stomach pains or diarrhoea after eating a cheese sandwich, try eating cheese on its own, or using a rice bread. Or stick to bread with a non-dairy filling. If orange juice seems to be problematic, try drinking it between meals, to rule out the possibility that it is another food causing the symptoms. The idea is not to eliminate the foods you regularly eat, but to avoid mixing them with other foods that may be possible offenders as well.

If, at the end of about a week or two, you are no nearer to isolating the offending foods, an elimination diet can be considered.

must know

Seeking medical help
If you suspect a food allergy or intolerance it is important to get proper medical advice – firstly to rule out any other illness, and secondly to get an accurate diagnosis. True food allergies, which usually provoke an immediate reaction, are generally straightforward to diagnose, but in most cases of food intolerance, identification can be more difficult.

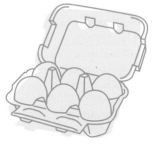

Changing your diet

On page 82, we look at eliminating foods for the purposes of both diagnosing which ones cause problems, but also as a tool for excluding problematic foods indefinitely – or at least until reintroduction is considered appropriate.

You can, however, undertake a very simple elimination test at home. Because a varied diet is so crucial to health and wellbeing, as it contains all of the nutrients we need to survive, you should never remove more than one suspected food at a time, and should also take steps to ensure that any nutrients that food contains are replaced. For example, cutting out cow's milk and dairy may leave your diet short of calcium, vitamin D and protein. These can easily be replaced by substituting other foods (see page 31). In the short term, it is not detrimental to be slightly short of some nutrients; in the long term, however, it can dramatically affect your health.

Experts suggest that randomly withdrawing foods from your child's diet can be dangerous, as it leaves it unbalanced at a time when nutrients are required for normal growth and development.

Make sure you undertake any changes under the supervision of a doctor or dietitian. An elimination diet should have a fairly immediate effect. Certainly in the case of sensitivities and intolerance you should notice that the symptoms are alleviated within a few days. Allergies can, of course, be multiple, so withdrawing one or two foods might not make a dramatic difference. In this case, you will

watch out!

Do not be tempted to reintroduce foods without checking that the allergy has disappeared. Even well-prepared people can be caught out by a severe reaction, and that's not a risk any of us would want to take.

need to have an assessment and tests undertaken by a trained professional – ideally an allergy specialist. Dropping foods from the diet is also, then, normally undertaken with the guidance of a dietitian, who can help ensure that your diet remains balanced.

Having said that, many people are intolerant to one food or food group, such as dairy, wheat or eggs. A short elimination diet will easily pinpoint this type of allergy, because the symptoms will reduce significantly. It is worth noting, however, that some experts claim that it can take up to two months for a food to entirely leave the body. So if you achieve short-term lessening of symptoms, but still do not feel a lot better, persevere for another few weeks. Food intolerances or sensitivities can be vast, or they can be limited to just one or two key foods, so try the foods you suspect one by one until you notice a difference.

In the case of suspected food allergies (dramatic symptoms, rather than niggling health complaints in most cases), do not attempt to reintroduce the food into your diet immediately. You will probably need to remove the danger food from your diet for a year or even more, after which your doctor will likely agree to a food challenge test (see page 87).

Diagnosis and tests

A dramatic reaction to any food will usually ensure that you're seen by an allergy specialist fairly quickly, who can confirm the diagnosis in a variety of ways. Less severe reactions can be tested at home first, by keeping a food diary and eliminating problematic foods from your diet. If you can't work out the foods

must know
Elimination at home
Remember that the vast majority of allergies centre around the 'big eight' foods, which include cow's milk, eggs, soya, wheat, peanuts, tree nuts and sesame, fish and shellfish. It is always worth considering these foods as potential allergens first, noting your reactions to these foods both in a food diary, and, if they appear problematic, removing them, one by one, from your diet. This simple type of home 'elimination' diet can often confirm allergies and intolerance, before a trip to the doctor is even necessary. Never, however, remove more than one or two foods at a time – not only because it will compromise your health, but it will also make the results of your home test unclear.

to which you are allergic, intolerant or even just sensitive, an allergy specialist will be able to make a diagnosis for you. The standard ways to test for allergies include skin-prick tests and blood tests. It is worth noting that there are no accurate tests for non-allergic forms of food intolerance. The only positive way to diagnose a food intolerance is a properly managed elimination diet.

The allergy assessment

Your allergy specialist (who may be known as an allergist or an immunologist) will begin by taking a 'case history', which involves looking at your medical history, from birth right through to the present day. Other factors which are taken into consideration include the health of other family members, including parents. Parents who suffer from asthma, hay fever or eczema, but not food allergies, are also more likely to have children with allergies, and a predilection for allergic health conditions, such as eczema. Several studies show that children of allergic parents are 75 per cent more likely to suffer from allergies themselves, so there is a strong genetic link. Age is another consideration, as allergies tend to rise from birth through to adolescence, and then fall.

Your specialist will enquire about the contents of the foods, the frequency, seasonality, severity and nature of the symptoms, and will ask about the amount of time that elapses between eating a food and any reaction. This is one reason why it is handy to keep a food

must know

Allergy specialists
You should see or be referred to an allergy specialist if:
• you have a diagnosed food allergy
• you have a limited diet as a result of perceived reactions to foods
• you have a family history of allergies and are pregnant; there are many preventative measures that can be taken to prevent allergies in babies (see page 178)
• you have experienced allergic symptoms (urticaria, swelling, itching, wheezing, or gastrointestinal responses, such as vomiting or diarrhoea) when eating or preparing foods
• you suffer from itching or burning in your mouth when eating food, in particular raw fruits and vegetables
• you are a baby with gastrointestinal symptoms, such as vomiting, diarrhoea, blood in the stool and poor growth, that cannot otherwise be explained

diary in advance of any appointment, so that you have this information at your fingertips.

Other health conditions will be considered, as some may mimic the symptoms of food allergy. In a nutshell, every aspect of health and diet will be considered when making an assessment. Remember that many cases of suspected food allergy are not actually allergies at all; for example, a reaction to caffeine in chocolate or coffee, or amines in red wine, all produce symptoms similar to those experienced in true food allergy, but are not in fact allergies. What's more, the majority of reactions are very prompt in true food allergy. While many people suffer from a delayed reaction, this may indicate that food is not the problem.

The minefield of possibilities is one reason why seeing a food allergy specialist is crucial. It can be virtually impossible for the average person to self-diagnose unless the symptoms are extreme and repeat themselves. Most specialists will also examine you physically, largely to rule out other health conditions, and note your weight and height.

Skin prick tests

Allergy skin prick tests are the first line of diagnosis, largely because they are cheap, safe and easy to perform. They may be helpful to determine which foods, if any, are triggering allergic symptoms. The idea is to gauge your reaction by introducing a small amount of the suspected substance/s into the top layer of your skin. If you are allergic to the food, a welt or 'weal' will be produced. The bigger the weal, the more severe your reaction and, of course, your allergy. Skin tests work by detecting any allergen-specific IgE – which explains why they are not always successful in picking up allergies that are non-IgE (see page 11) mediated – such as many food intolerances.

Many specialists undertake skin prick tests in their offices, and they are safe and virtually painless. They can be used on patients of all ages, including young children, although the results in babies less than 12 months of age tend to be less reliable, as their skin is not as reactive. People suffering from skin conditions, such as eczema, are not usually good candidates for skin prick testing, and will have blood tests (see page 79) instead.

Skin prick tests are usually done on the inside of your forearm, although in young children, it may be done on their backs so they don't have to see what is happening. While the tests are not painful, it can be distressing or frightening to see what amounts to a tiny incision being made in your skin.

Most doctors begin by producing a 'test weal', which involves pricking the skin and putting a little histamine on the site. Histamine is the substance produced by the body when it comes into contact with an allergen. By pricking it directly into the skin, the body should react by producing a weal. The size of this weal is used to measure the severity of the other substances tested, but it can also indicate if there is any suppression of symptoms which may be caused by medication you are taking.

Next, a series of small pricks are made into the top layer of the skin (which does not cause any bleeding or bruising), and a small amount of the suspected allergen, in pure liquid form, is put in the site. In most cases your doctor will have the liquid form of your suspected allergen available, but sometimes you may be asked to bring in a fresh sample of the food itself.

A positive reaction to the skin prick test occurs when the skin around the needle prick becomes itchy and red with the development of a weal. The weal reaches its maximum size in about 15 to 20 minutes and the reaction fades within a few hours. The larger the weal, the more likely that you are to be allergic.

The allergens that will be tested are usually those to which you have expressed concern, although your specialist may also test other foods in the same group, other common foods (from the 'big eight' for example), or anything else that appears possible.

If the results are conclusive, you may not require a

must know

Allergy testing
It is very important that you do not take any of your usual allergy medication before skin-prick or blood testing, such as steroids, antihistamines or bronchodilators. These can mask your response to the allergens, and make the results unreliable. You should also tell your doctor if you have been ill, are suffering from any illness, or have or are taking a course of antibiotics. These factors too can affect the results of tests.

blood test, although many specialists will offer one to confirm the diagnosis, and to test for other possible foods. A wider number of allergens can be tested using your blood.

Blood tests

This test, called a RAST (radio-allergosorbent test), measures the antibodies in your bloodstream to certain food allergens. The test may also be called a 'Cap-RAST' test; they are the same thing. For this type of test, a sample of your blood is taken and sent to a specialist laboratory. The RAST measures the amount of specific Immunoglobulin E antibodies (IgE, which trigger a histamine release) in your blood to various food allergens. So if you are allergic to wheat, your 'wheat IgE' will be raised. The test can be undertaken for different parts of the wheat, such as gluten, and the whole wheat grain.

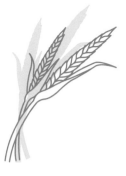

The result is then graded 0 to 6, depending on the level of that particular IgE in the blood. A low grade, say 1 or 2, may suggest a milder allergy; in some instances people suffering from mild allergies are able to tolerate small amounts of the food without any real problem, and are also more likely to outgrow them. It is still recommended that you avoid these foods for a period of time (for milder allergies, between three months and a year), after which the tests can be repeated to check your status.

Over 400 different allergens can be tested for in this way (this number includes environmental allergens as well, such as pollens, moulds and even dust mites). Your specialist may take the opportunity to test for some of these environmental allergens at the same time.

Unlike the skin prick test, a RAST test has a high degree of false negatives, meaning it may not detect food allergies that you really have. A positive RAST test is a reliable indicator that you are likely to be allergic to that food. If a certain food, such as peanuts, shows up positive on a RAST test, it means you are more likely than not to be allergic to that food. If a skin test and a RAST test agree, you can give the results even more weight. It is also important to remember that other factors can affect the results. Once again, if you have been ill or are rundown, if there is anti-allergy medication circulating in your bloodstream, or you have recently taken antibiotics, the results may not be accurate. Similarly, if it is hay fever season and you are suffering badly, you may become more sensitive to suspect foods – largely because your body is in overdrive and all allergic reactions are heightened. So a strong result during this period may not be fully accurate. That's why taking a full medical history is so important – the timing of symptoms and 'attacks' may reflect other factors causing or exacerbating symptoms. Food allergies are still not fully understood by the medical profession, although ongoing research has improved the position over the last decade.

Food challenge tests

If the diagnosis of food allergy remains in doubt, your doctor may recommend a food challenge test. These tests are conducted in the doctor's office, or, if a serious reaction is feared, in the hospital under close observation.

Usually, the suspected food or a neutral food, called a placebo, is fed to the patient in colourless capsules, or in a non-allergenic food, such as broth. Neither the patient nor the doctor knows whether the suspected food or the placebo is being eaten.

must know

Skin prick tests
Blood tests will be undertaken on their own, without a skin prick test, in very young children, eczema or other skin condition sufferers, and in anyone with a history of life-threatening reactions to food substances. For example, few doctors would risk a peanut skin prick test if there is a risk of anaphylaxis. Some sufferers are so sensitive that even being in the same room as the offending food can cause a serious reaction.

This type of food challenge is called a 'double-blind' challenge, which basically means that neither you nor your doctor knows what you are taking, and you will be given a placebo or 'dummy' food some of the time. In most cases, it involves giving you increasing amounts of the problem food over about three hours, in order to see the response. You may be kept in the doctor's surgery, clinic or hospital for up to a day so that the reactions can be properly gauged. Because life-threatening reactions are usually instant, you will not normally have to stay overnight for observation (unless, of course, you have suffered a response).

Sometimes shorter 'open challenges' are performed where the patient is aware of what they are eating. The same agenda is observed, however, with increasing amounts offered over a period of time until a reaction is obvious – or none recorded.

Some reactions, particularly in the case of intolerance, can show up even 48 hours later, but in most cases you will have a follow-up appointment to discuss reactions.

When properly performed, these challenges are very reliable in establishing a concrete cause and effect relationship between a food and an allergy symptom. Many people also feel safer testing food in the safety of a doctor's surgery or hospital setting. A food challenge test may also be used to 'retest' foods to which you have been allergic in the past, and which you may now have outgrown.

Only one food is challenged at a time, and if tolerated, you are given a plan and instructions on how to continue at home. For multiple allergies, a number of repeat visits may be necessary.

must know
Repeat testing
Once allergies have been identified through one or more of the tests noted in this chapter, you will be under the care of an allergy specialist and often a dietitian, who can help you to replace missing nutrients in your diet to ensure that it is well balanced. This is particularly important for children. Tests will be repeated, often on a six-monthly basis, especially in the case of children who tend to outgrow allergies, to see if the food is still a problem. Long-term allergies in adults will not, however, usually be re-tested unless you have cause to think they are no longer present.

The elimination diet

An elimination diet is one of the best ways to diagnose a food allergy or intolerance. It must be properly managed, followed by a food challenge, and used alongside a food diary to be most effective.

There are several different ways to go about an elimination diet. A simple diet, to pinpoint a problematic food (see page 84) can be undertaken at home, and will almost always confirm foods to which you are allergic. This is one of the most accurate ways to pinpoint food intolerance. Blood tests and skin prick tests may fail to pick food intolerances up, because they do not involve an allergic reaction (IgE).

The most effective diagnostic test for food intolerance is to remove all potentially offending foods from the diet for up to two weeks. If the symptoms resolve on this elimination diet, then generally a diagnosis of food intolerance can be made. Such an elimination diet should not be attempted without dietetic and medical supervision, as the diet is restrictive and may not be nutritionally adequate.

Confirmation of the diagnosis of food intolerance and subsequent identification of the problem food is then achieved by gradually re-introducing individual foods or food chemicals into the diet in increasing doses over several days. If a reaction occurs, the food is withdrawn from the diet again, and the symptoms allowed to clear before another food or food chemical is tested.

Once the foods and food chemicals to which you are intolerant have been identified, the next step is to establish the dose and frequency with which the problem foods can be safely eaten. Unlike food allergy, where complete avoidance of the food(s) is usually necessary, most people can tolerate some amount of the food or chemicals to which they are intolerant. Symptoms are prevented by avoiding a build-up of the food chemicals in the body over several days.

In Chapter Five, we'll look at allergies in children. The elimination diet is undertaken in a different way for children, so don't be tempted to adapt an adult exclusion diet if you suspect your child has allergies.

Some specialists advise removing just one food at a time from your diet, and then reintroducing it; however, this is not practical if you fear multiple allergies or intolerances, as it can take many months to achieve a realistic diagnosis. Furthermore, you may still experience symptoms from the foods you *are* eating, and to which you may also be allergic, so losing one food from your diet for several weeks, even if it is known to be an allergen, may not make any dramatic difference to the way you feel.

The best way to proceed is to undertake what is known as the 'few foods' diet. This basically means removing all foods that could cause allergy from your diet, and relying instead upon a quite strict diet for several weeks. You will need to look carefully at the list of 'acceptable' foods, because some may well be triggers for you. If you suspect one to be problematic, leave it out. A few foods diet should not continue for more than two weeks.

Preparing for the diet

You will need to be extremely strict about your eating habits for the next four to six weeks, so empty your cupboards of anything that might tempt you off your diet, and make sure you stock up on all the foods that will be required to keep you from snacking on the wrong foods. There can be no 'cheating' on an elimination diet, as you will not achieve a firm diagnosis. Many experts also recommend that you take a vitamin and mineral supplement while undergoing an elimination diet. Look for a brand that does not contain yeast, gelatine or nut oils. You will want to ensure that it also contains plenty of calcium and vitamin B, which will most likely be lacking on this diet.

Stage one: healthy eating

Before embarking on a simple or strict elimination diet, ensure you eat healthy foods for two weeks. This simply involves eating fresh, unprocessed foods, avoiding additives, preservatives and other chemicals in food that may be clouding the picture in relation to your allergies. Many people find that when they remove processed foods and 'junk' foods and drinks from their diet, their symptoms are reduced or even disappear altogether. The reasons for this are many, but it may just be that you are sensitive to one or more chemicals in foods. During this period, you should eat whole grains wherever possible (there are many chemicals added to grains when they are refined), a wide variety of fresh fruit and vegetables (organic if possible, as this reduces the risk of pesticide and sulphite exposure, or sulphites (see page 60), fresh fish, poultry and meat, plenty of rice, good-quality oils, such as olive oil, fresh dairy produce, and pulses (legumes). If you are not sensitive to nuts and seeds, include these as they are a good way to add protein and healthy oils. Avoid coffee, tea, soft drinks, processed foods, crisps, baked goods, alcohol – in short anything that comes in a 'packet'.

You may find that changing your diet to one that is healthier makes all the difference. Food allergies may not actually be a problem for you. If, however, you do not notice a dramatic difference, and you are still experiencing symptoms in response to eating one or more foods, you will need to move on to a simple elimination diet.

Stage two: simple elimination

Carry on with the healthy eating programme, but remove the foods that you suspect cause problems. If you suspect more than one food, remove them all from your diet. After a period of two or three weeks, you can reintroduce them, one by one. Start with small quantities, and note any symptoms, gradually increasing to a full 'portion'. If you don't have any problems, add back another food, and gauge your response. Take care to read labels very carefully. Ingesting even small quantities of offending foods, which may appear as ingredients in

Cravings

Cravings are one of the key symptoms of food intolerance. Some studies show that at least 50 per cent of us suffer food cravings for problem foods. We may even be unaware of it. Take a look at your own diet and see what foods you eat most commonly. Try cutting out these foods for several weeks and see if you experience better health to any significant degree. Many people who suffer from regular headaches, low-grade niggling health problems and fatigue are intolerant or sensitive to certain foods, and it is not until these foods are removed that they become aware that a problem exists. Look at the foods your child chooses, particularly if she is a picky eater. Children who refuse to eat anything other than peanut butter sandwiches, or pasta and cereal, show clear-cut tendencies for suspect foods.

When you go on an elimination diet, your body may go through withdrawal symptoms, triggering cravings for the very food that is not good for it. In a nutshell, our body doesn't always know what is right for it! So a craving can be an important symptom to note. Withdrawal symptoms can be quite fierce for a few days, and may involve tearfulness, irritability, fatigue, headaches and shakiness. If they persist for longer than three or four days, see your doctor.

other food items, can render the elimination diet largely ineffective, as symptoms will continue, particularly if you are very sensitive.

It is worth noting, too, that you can often feel much worse on an elimination diet, and this feeling of malaise can continue for up to six days. As a rule of thumb, the sixth or seventh day is the point at which you rebound and, if food really is the problem, experience a significant improvement in symptoms and overall wellbeing.

All elimination diets, whether they are simple or more extensive, should be undertaken with the help of a doctor or dietitian. Even small changes to your diet can mean that you are missing out on key nutrients, and nutritional imbalances can affect your health on many levels.

Stage three: strict exclusion diet

A full elimination diet, or strict exclusion diet, must only be followed with the advice of a dietitian or qualified doctor, as serious nutritional deficiencies are a real risk. The idea is to stick to the 'few foods' diet

must know

The 'few foods' diet
The following foods are considered to have a low potential for causing allergies, and will form the basis of a strict exclusion diet:
Meat: lamb, chicken
Vegetables: rice, sweet potato, carrots, rhubarb, asparagus
Fruit: pears, banana, apricots, apple, pineapple (all peeled)
Fat: non-dairy margarine, sunflower and olive oil
Other: herbal tea, water, honey, sugar, sago
Herbs and spices are generally OK, but use them sparingly, and avoid anything that has triggered a reaction in the past.

(choosing eight to ten of the least allergenic foods), which means eating a fairly bland, strict diet for a period of ten to 14 days. Many people find this type of diet boring and difficult to manage, as eating out is tricky, and the foods allowed can be very limiting. Don't be misled into thinking that staying on the diet for longer than 14 days is appropriate. Nutritional depletion on the 'few foods' diet can, after two weeks, lead to the suppression of your immune system. So it may appear that your 'over-responsive' immune system is no longer over-reacting to foods, but in fact, it is merely suppressed due to nutritional deficiency. When a normal diet begins again, the immune system is reactivated and the symptoms recur. In addition, other foods that were previously tolerated may appear to be problematic.

Stick only to these foods considered to be low allergen (see page 141), and reduce the list still further if you suspect one of these foods to be problematic. You can adapt these foods to some degree, for more variety. For example, rice pasta, rice cakes or even rice noodles make a change from plain rice, and you can cook using a vegan stock, adding acceptable fruits and vegetables to meats to create tasty dishes. Vegan stock can also be used to make simple soups (see page 91). Don't fill your diet with 'allergy-free' alternatives, such as 'non-wheat' breads or biscuits. The idea is to streamline your diet as much as possible, and many of these goods have long lists of ingredients that could be a potential source of allergy. Only the foods on this list are acceptable. Avoid alcohol, tea and coffee; herbal teas are usually acceptable, although there is some evidence that teas such as chamomile can trigger symptoms in hay fever sufferers. Water and diluted fruit juices are your best bet.

Reintroduction after strict elimination

Once the allergy has settled after four to eight weeks on the elimination diet, other foods are slowly reintroduced one at a time at weekly intervals. Each new food may be tried in small test quantities and then given in normal amounts every day for a week until the allergy-provoking food is identified. Most foods can then slowly be reintroduced during the provocation testing period. Slowly reintroduce fish and shellfish, pork and beef, nuts, chocolate, legumes (pulses), white potatoes, tomatoes, oranges, strawberries, cow's milk, wheat, eggs, pizza, fresh fruit and finally hen's eggs. Provocation testing should not be performed if there is a history of anaphylaxis to a particular food (such as peanuts or shellfish). In this case, any reintroduction will be undertaken under the guidance of a trained professional.

Should you suffer any reaction to a food upon reintroduction, drop it again and wait a few days before introducing another food. Most experts recommend that if a food causes problems upon reintroduction, it should be removed from your diet for at least six months before trying it again. Once again, only try foods that do not provoke a life-threatening reaction.

As a tool for diagnosing food allergies and intolerance, an elimination diet can be invaluable. In the next chapter we will look at how to manage a food allergy once it has been diagnosed.

must know
Exclusion for life
There is no doubt that some foods will continue to be problematic, and it may well be that you suffer from a life-long allergy. One or two food allergies can be easy to manage; however, multiple allergies can threaten your nutritional status because you will have to avoid a number of food groups for an extended period of time. In the next chapter we'll look at ways to make this easier, and to ensure that you are getting the nutrients you need. It is essential that you get the help of a dietitian or nutritionist to help balance your diet. You will also need to become adept at reading labels, as even small quantities of offending foods can cause and/or exacerbate the symptoms, and prevent the likelihood of outgrowing the allergy.

Cooking on an elimination diet

It is not as difficult as you might think to create nutritious, healthy meals based on a limited number of foods. Casseroles, soups and stews using fruit, vegetables, meat and vegan stock are delicious and filling, and they also ensure that you get good levels of key nutrients. Here are some ideas for meals on the 'few foods' diet.

Other ideas

Roast carrots with a little honey and sea salt, until just tender and lightly browned. Serve with chicken, lamb or rice.

Honey roasted chicken and sweet potato

Serves 2

2 chicken breasts
Runny honey
Olive oil
2 sweet potatoes, peeled and cut into 'chips'
Salt and pepper

Simply drizzle honey and olive oil over the chicken breasts and sweet potato chips. Season to taste. Place chicken breasts on the sweet potato, on a non-stick pan, and cook at 180°C/350°F/Gas 4 degrees for about 30 minutes, or until chicken is tender and lightly browned. Add a light salad of lettuce, grated carrots and grated apple, drizzled with olive oil and a little honey, for a balanced meal.

Other ideas

Make sweet potato 'chips' by drizzling them with olive oil, a little salt and pepper, and roasting at 220°C/425°F/Gas 7 until lightly browned. Serve as a side dish or on their own.

Moroccan lamb and apricot tagine

Serves 4

2 tbsp olive oil

4 strands of saffron

$1/2$ tsp ground turmeric (avoid if you have had any sensitivity to spices in the past)

$1/2$ tsp ground black pepper

$1/2$ tsp ground ginger

$1/2$ tsp cayenne pepper

675g/1-$1/2$lb lamb, cut into large cubes

Water

300g/11oz dried apricots (without sulphur dioxide; choose fresh, peeled apricots if you can't find them)

450g/1lb sweet potatoes, peeled and cut into 5-cm/2-in. pieces

90ml/3fl oz honey

90ml/3fl oz water

1 x 2.5-cm/1-in. cinnamon stick

In a large bowl, mix together the oil, saffron, turmeric, pepper, ginger, cayenne until well blended. Add the meat and toss to coat.

Heat a large casserole or saucepan over moderately high heat until hot then add the meat and sear on all sides. Add enough water so the meat is just covered, bring to a boil, then reduce the heat, cover and simmer for 1 hour and 45 minutes.

Add the apricots, mix well then raise the heat a little and cook, uncovered, until the sauce is reduced to about 240ml/8fl oz.

Meanwhile, place the sweet potato, honey, water and cinnamon stick in a saucepan. Bring to the boil then reduce the heat and simmer for 15 minutes.

Reduce the sweet potato cooking liquor by boiling rapidly until syrupy. Add the sweet potato mixture to the meat and its juice, mixing well, then simmer for a further 5 minutes. Serve hot with rice.

Other ideas

Bake a sweet potato as you would a jacket potato, and drizzle with olive oil and salt and pepper.

Other ideas

- Roast a chicken at the beginning of the week, and use the leftovers for salads with grated carrots, lettuce and cooked rice, teamed with a light honey, olive oil and thyme dressing. Use the juices as the basis for a stock (added to a vegan stock powder) or to flavour other foods. Or make your own by stewing the bones for several hours with two carrots, a bay leaf, a leek and a cubed sweet potato. Use shredded chicken to enhance other meals.
- Baked pears, pineapple or bananas, cooked in foil with a little brown sugar, honey and vanilla, are a quick and delicious standby for dessert.

Baked asparagus risotto

Serves 4

1 tbsp olive oil
2 leeks, sliced (not strictly on the diet, but usually fine for most sufferers)
1 tbsp thyme leaves
300g/11oz arborio rice
750ml/26fl oz vegan stock
800g/1lb 12oz asparagus, sliced

Preheat the oven to 200°C/400°F/Gas 6. Heat a frying pan over high heat. Add the oil, leeks and thyme, and cook for 5 minutes, or until the leeks are lightly browned. Spoon the mixture into a 4-pint capacity ovenproof dish. Add the rice and stock, and stir. Season to taste. Cover tightly with aluminium foil and bake for 20 minutes. Add the asparagus, re-cover, and bake for a further 20 minutes. Remove the risotto from the oven, add further salt and pepper as required, and stir until the risotto has absorbed all the liquid. This recipe is good as a main course or side dish.

You can adapt this dish by adding two chicken breasts, cubed, to the first stage of the recipe, lightly browning them with the leeks and olive oil.

Other ideas

Be inventive! Team fruit with meat (as they do in many parts of Europe and Northern Africa). For example, bananas, chicken and apricots make a delicious combination served with rice.

Carrot and coriander soup

Serves 4

1.5 litres/2 pints water (or vegan stock)
500g/1lb carrots, peeled and chopped
2 medium sweet potatoes, peeled and chopped
2 leeks, sliced
1 dessertspoon sunflower or olive oil
Small bunch of fresh coriander
Salt and pepper to taste

In a large saucepan, bring water (or vegan stock) to a boil. Add carrots and sweet potatoes and simmer with the lid on the pan. In a separate frying pan, gently cook leeks for about 8 minutes, in sunflower or olive oil, or until they are soft and lightly browned, but not crispy.

Add the contents of the pan to the carrots. Leave the soup to cook on a moderate heat and chop coriander finely. When the carrots and potatoes are soft, transfer the mix to a blender or food processor, and whiz until smooth. Add salt and pepper to taste, and, if necessary, a little dried vegan stock powder (to add a little lift).

Return to the saucepan, and stir in the coriander. Let it simmer for a few minutes. Serve with tiny leek matchsticks and coriander on top. This also makes a good 'sauce' for rice noodles. For variety, add leftover roasted chicken breast or rice.

Other ideas

• Lamb shoulder, lightly browned and oven-cooked slowly in apricot or apple juice, is delicious served hot with rice noodles or fresh white rice. A little salt and pepper is all you'll need!
• Make a big mixed fruit salad for breakfasts or puddings. Top with freshly chopped mint or drizzle with honey if you like things a little sweeter. Top rice cakes with a little honey or margarine to serve on the side.

Other tests

There are an increasing number of allergy tests now available, due to the fact that food allergies have become more prominent in recent years. It must be stressed that by far the most reliable tests are those that have been described previously in this chapter; and, when all else fails, an exclusion diet will pinpoint anything that may slip through the orthodox testing net.

While many of the 'new' tests are based on valid principles, others are simply not effective and may cause you to eliminate foods from your diet unnecessarily, which can undermine both your health and quality of life. Before you undertake any of the tests described below, do ensure that you are working with a registered, experienced practitioner who will explain how it works, and give some examples of its efficacy.

Some of the alternative testing listed below has merited some good research, with equally good results. Others are simple quackery, and should not be considered.

watch out!

Home-testing kits are expensive and often unreliable. If you do decide to purchase one, do not eliminate anything from your diet until you have consulted a trained allergy specialist, who you can normally be referred to by your doctor. Anyone with a full-blown 'true' allergy will be aware of foods that cause problems, and cases of intolerance and sensitivities are best investigated through a sensible exclusion diet or tests arranged by your doctor.

VEGA testing

This involves measuring 'disordered' electromagnetic current in your body. This test was developed by German doctor Reinhold Voll in 1958, so although it is certainly well established in terms of longevity, it must be said that many (including the British Medical Journal) view it as being of dubious use. Also called the 'electrodermal test', VEGA uses a 'wheatstone bridge galvanometer' to measure electromagnetic conductivity in the body. An electrode is placed over an acupuncture point, and another electrode is held while various allergens are placed in a metallic device. If there is a fall in electromagnetic conductivity, or a change in the reading, it indicates an intolerance or allergy to that substance. This system has been updated into computerized versions of the same technique, which are quicker to diagnose. There have been several studies undertaken to investigate the validity of this test; however, the results have not been promising.

Applied kinesiology

This is an interesting one. Applied kinesiology tests muscle strength in the presence of various allergens. A loss of strength is reported to indicate an allergy. The science of applied kinesiology was developed in the early 1960s in the US, and relies on energy fields within the body. Phials of allergic substances are placed, one by one, in front of the sufferer. He or she holds out an arm and the practitioner applies counter pressure. If she is not able to resist the counter pressure, the test is considered to be positive to that allergy. The antidote to the allergy is then held in front of the sufferer, and if their weakness is reversed, it indicates that it is the correct antidote. There are a number of variations to the technique of muscle testing and many practitioners also use magnets. The British Society for Allergy and Clinical Immunology has found this test unreliable. However, there is a great body of followers, and some claim that it is up to 95 per cent accurate.

Hair analysis

The idea behind hair analysis is that it shows up mineral deficiencies (such as selenium, zinc, chromium, manganese and magnesium), which are believed to indicate an allergy. Some practitioners also test for the presence of heavy metals, such as mercury and lead, although the link between these substances and allergies is not clearly defined.

A sample of your hair, from close to the scalp (not a cutting), if possible, is taken and sent to a laboratory. Most analysis is now done by computer, and some 'reports' can be extensive (and potentially very misleading). Certainly hair analysis can indicate some deficiencies in some patients, and is valuable in testing for heavy metal exposure, but as a tool for diagnosing

must know
Desensitization
Many untrained practitioners offer not only diagnostic techniques which may be suspect, but also desensitization programmes. Desensitization involves injecting progressively larger doses of a food so that the body becomes less sensitive, and stops reacting. While desensitization may work for hay fever and other allergies related to inhaled substances, it is worthless for foods and can be dangerous.

allergies, it is not considered to be reliable. For one thing, shampoos, environmental pollutants, and hair dyes can affect the mineral content of hair; what's more, there is no clear link between mineral deficiencies and specific food allergies. A study published in 2001 concluded that hair mineral analysis from labs was unreliable.

Provocation-neutralization

This procedure involves testing a sufferer with a small amount of allergenic substance in liquid form – either injected into the skin, or offered in drop form (the normal way; which is placed under the tongue). Ten minutes after the test, the patient is then asked to record any symptoms, no matter how mild. A 'positive' result is said to be achieved if *any* symptoms are experienced. If the patient fails to report a symptom, the test is repeated using the same substance at a different concentration until there is a 'positive' result. Next, the same substance is tested at lower concentrations until the patient again fails to report a symptom, at which point the allergy (the symptom) is said to be 'neutralized'. The neutralizing dose of the substance is then prescribed as a form of treatment. Each substance has to be tested separately, which means that the process is very time consuming. Moreover, several studies have found that patients react equally to placebo (dummy injections or drops), which means that the results are pretty much useless. The American Academy of Allergy and Immunology says no controlled studies demonstrate either diagnostic or therapeutic effects.

Cytotoxic Food Testing - ALCAT

The cytotoxic test for food allergy consists of applying one drop of diluted whole blood to a microscope slide that was previously coated with a dry film of a food extract. The slide is examined microscopically for swelling, collapse or other distortion of white blood cells. Any such change indicates a food allergy to the offending substance. These tests are also known as 'leucocytotoxic tests' and the 'Nutron' test. According to the European Academy for Allergology and Clinical Immunology. All of these tests had a poor reliability for diagnosing allergies when they were subjected to trials according to the European Academy for Allergology and Clinical Immunology.

ELISA/ACT

Another allergy test of questionable accuracy is IgG ELISA/ACT test. This test measures IgG antibodies to various foods. While this may sound similar to the UniCAP or RAST tests, there is an important difference. RAST tests for IgE antibodies, which are those that the body produces in the case of true allergy. ELISA tests for IgG antibodies. Studies show that most people develop IgG antibodies to foods they eat and this is a normal response indicating exposure but not sensitization. Once again, no clear evidence exists to say that ELISA successfully diagnoses allergies. Some sceptics claim that because dietary/nutritional advice is usually offered afterwards, it is simply a means by which further and often unnecessary treatment can be offered by less orthodox health practitioners. Furthermore, this test can now be purchased for home use, so there is an added element of sales motivation involved here. Plus, of course, there is great scope for misdiagnosis, and subsequently a nutritionally weak diet.

watch out!

Even small doses of allergens used for test purposes can cause a life-threatening reaction in susceptible people. Many practitioners offering alternative allergy testing techniques are not equipped to deal with medical emergencies. If you have ever experienced a serious reaction to any food, do not undertake these tests unless under the care of a registered health practitioner.

Iridology

Iridology is also known as 'iris diagnosis', and it is based on the premise that a corresponding area of the iris in the eye represents an area of the body. The idea is that overall health and sites of disease can be diagnosed from the colour, texture and location of various flecks of pigment in the iris. This practice has many followers, and many claim that illnesses relating to specific organs have been successfully diagnosed through studying the iris, but it is difficult to see how this could be used to diagnose any food allergies.

Case study

Freddie

Freddie was two when he began to react to different foods – suffering skin rashes around his mouth when he ate eggs or dairy produce, vomiting when he ate fish, and experiencing wheezing when he ate anything containing tree nuts. He was an allergic child, with eczema that was controlled by steroids, and tended to suffer from asthmatic symptoms whenever he had a cold. His doctor referred him to an allergy specialist, who asked his parents to keep a diary of all foods he ate, and note any reactions, as well as the timing of when these reactions occurred. They discovered that his regular fussiness at bedtime was almost always the result of his evening bottle of formula milk being offered, and also found that even small amounts of egg made his eczema instantly worse.

He was offered a skin prick test for seven foods, and these tests, despite his young age, were undertaken on his forearm. Because the procedure is largely painless, he was not distressed by the testing, and was distracted by a play therapist at the hospital while his specialist did the tests. After a 15-minute wait, his skin was checked to see how large the weals were. It was clear that cod, tree nuts, cow's milk and egg white were all strong contenders, while egg yolk, soya and wheat showed little or no reaction.

Freddie was also given a RAST blood test, in which further foods were tested alongside the original seven. He found the blood tests uncomfortable, and was distressed by the procedure. He returned to the hospital with his parents three weeks later to discuss the results, which confirmed what the skin prick tests suggested – he had a strong allergy to cod, tree nuts, cow's milk and egg white, and also to peanuts. Minor sensitivities to other foods were noted.

He was then placed in the hands of a dietitian, who helped his parents ensure that both his calorific and nutritional needs were being met. Milk was replaced with soya and hydrolyzed formulas; fish was removed from the diet, as were eggs and all nuts, including peanuts. A calcium supplement was prescribed, as well as a general multivitamin and mineral syrup. Freddie's overall health improved immediately. His eczema virtually disappeared, although occasionally resurfaced when suspect foods were accidentally eaten. His evening fussiness and regular bouts of diarrhoea and vomiting were also a thing of the past. His mother also arranged for him to see a homeopath, to work on increasing his basic immunity, so that his system did not continue to over-react to the same extent. To the delight of his parents and the consultant, who he saw every six months, Freddie outgrew all of his allergies by the age of five, although large quantities of milk still cause some discomfort.

want to know more?

For further information on tests, where they can be offered both within and outside the NHS, as well as general information on food allergies, visit Action against Allergy: www.actionagainstallergy.co.uk.

Set up by the parents of two allergic sons, the allergy site gives free information about all major allergies. It lists symptoms, triggers and treatment. Also featured are support forums, allergen info, useful numbers, testing, links and product information. Visit www.theallergysite.co.uk.

The magazine Foods Matter is the UK's only periodical for those suffering from food allergies, sensitivities and intolerance, or anyone on a restricted diet. Visit www.foodsmatter.com for details.

While home testing is not usually a good idea, York Nutritional Laboratory offers a good service, with kits and information packs, as well as an excellent site with guidance on food allergy and intolerance. They have a good follow-up service with sensible advice. If you can't get any response from your GP, try: www.allergy-testing.com

The Food Allergy Initiative offers information, advice and lots more; visit www.foodallergyinitiative.org.

4 Managing your allergies

Allergic reactions to food can range from being slight or simply annoying to severe and even life-threatening. However, symptoms can be controlled by adopting an allergen-free lifestyle, being aware of symptoms in the event that you do accidentally eat problematic foods, and knowing how to treat your symptoms. In the case of life-threatening allergies you will need to administer emergency treatment.

Allergic reactions

In Chapter One, we looked at some of the main symptoms that food allergies can cause. However, because each person tends to react in very individual ways, it is important that you learn to recognize your own symptoms.

Your food diary (see page 72) will help you to pinpoint the key responses you may have to suspect foods. For example, many people with allergies suffer an instant rash around the mouth, a burning sensation on the lips, hives, itching – and, more dramatically – breathing problems or vomiting. But again, sometimes symptoms can take time to manifest themselves, and may not even appear until a day or two later. Recognizing your own pattern of response will make things much easier. You may find, for example, that you can tolerate small quantities of suspect foods, but that larger ones are more problematic. Knowledge is power, so take the time to become as self-aware as you can.

must know

Oral allergy syndrome

This is an instant type of reaction to specific foods, which affect the mouth and throat - rather like contact dermatitis, but in the mouth. You may develop a sensation of itching or tingling of the lips, tongue, palate, and throat after eating certain foods. In addition, your lips and tongue may swell, and your throat may feel tight. This is often the first sign of a reaction for many sufferers.

For example, if you are aware that cow's milk causes digestive discomfort about 48 hours after consumption, you can check your diet two days earlier to see how you may have come to eat or drink something containing milk or dairy produce. If your reactions tend to be more immediate to some foods, you can work out the offending item fairly quickly and stop eating at once. Similarly, becoming aware of your unique symptoms – a tingling mouth, for example – means that you can be prepared for the next stage, and take the appropriate medication.

Food allergies are far less stressful and debilitating if you know yourself and your own reactions.

Anaphylaxis

We looked at this serious condition briefly in Chapter One, and anyone who has experienced anaphylaxis as a result of eating a food to which they are allergic should always be prepared for emergency treatment.

Anaphylaxis is a sudden, severe, potentially fatal allergic reaction that can involve various areas of the body, such as the skin, respiratory tract, gastrointestinal tract and/or heart and lungs. In most cases, this reaction sets in just moments after eating the problem food; however, it can be two hours and – rarely – up to four hours before symptoms set in. It is, therefore, crucial that you are prepared at all times.

An anaphylactic reaction may begin with a tingling sensation, itching, or metallic taste in the mouth. Other symptoms can include hives, a sensation of warmth, asthma symptoms, swelling of the mouth and throat area, difficulty breathing, vomiting, diarrhoea, cramping, a drop in blood pressure, and loss of consciousness. As it may take a couple of hours for these symptoms to develop fully, it is extremely important that you are aware of the first signs – which are, in many cases, flushing, breathing problems, and a strange taste or tingling in your mouth.

In some people, something called a 'biphasic' reaction can occur. In this cases symptoms appear to resolve, and then return again several hours later.

> **must know**
> **Anaphylaxis action**
> The Food Allergy and Anaphylaxis Network suggest the 'three Rs' for treating anaphylaxis. These are:
> • recognize symptoms
> • react quickly
> • review what happened and be sure to prevent it from recurring

Treating anaphylaxis

The most important, immediate, treatment is to reverse the symptoms as soon as possible. Epinephrine (which is adrenaline) is the drug most often

watch out!

Your life may be saved by remembering the following:

- always advise your doctor if you experience a serious reaction to any food
- always act quickly. Never assume you have time to waste
- always carry your medication – an EpiPen or whatever your doctor has prescribed
- if this is your first attack or you are not carrying your medication, call for an ambulance immediately
- if you are eating food that you have not prepared, make sure that everyone you are with knows about your allergy, and what should be done in an emergency
- your friends and families family should all be aware of what you need to avoid, how to recognize the symptoms, and how to administer treatment
- wear a medic alert bracelet to advise others of your allergy
- all cases of anaphylaxis should be seen in hospital, whether medication has been effective or not

prescribed for this purpose. Your doctor or allergy specialist can prescribe epinephrine, which is available in the form of an EpiPen, which you use to inject yourself (or, in the case of younger children, or the later stages of an attack, is injected by someone else).

Adrenaline (epinephrine) works directly on the heart and lungs, countering the effects of anaphylaxis. It relaxes the muscles in the lungs to improve breathing, reverses swelling and stimulates the heartbeat.

An EpiPen is an automatic injection device that will deliver one single dose of adrenaline. It can be given through clothing and, once used, cannot be reused. You may need to carry two pens to be safe. If the first dose is not enough, it can be repeated within five to ten minutes. It is extremely important that you carry your EpiPen with you at all times.

Antihistamines and steroids may also be taken in an attack, to ease swelling, breathing difficulties and other symptoms. These are taken alongside epinephrine, never instead of it, as they will help recovery, but will not reverse symptoms that can, unchecked, lead to death. Some sufferers may recognize the early symptoms of a food reaction, in the form of flushing or a burning mouth, for example, and instantly taking an antihistamine will avoid a full-blown attack of anaphylaxis. However, symptoms must be caught immediately in order for antihistamine to have a significant effect. Similarly, steroids can improve breathing in the early stages of an attack, but must be taken quickly to be effective.

Emergency treatment

It's not just enough to be aware of the early signs of anaphylaxis. Some people suffering their first severe reaction may not be aware of the severity of their condition, and fail to respond appropriately. It's only on second and subsequent occasions that they realize that emergency treatment is required.

There are several important things to consider here. The first is that getting food allergies properly diagnosed is crucial to successful treatment. Any dramatic reaction to a food has the potential to lead to anaphylaxis in susceptible people. For example, asthmatics are more likely to respond in this way to serious allergies. Moreover, some people become increasingly sensitized to problem food each time it is eaten, which means that subsequent reactions can be more and more extreme. Your doctor or specialist will be able to diagnose a serious allergy, by the details you give him or her, as well as through the various tests offered. They will also recommend an immediate course of treatment, and usually provide prescriptions for an EpiPen, and perhaps other drugs (see page 104).

Secondly, you may experience an immediate dramatic reaction to a food, without recognizing the early symptoms. In this case, it is important that you wear a medic alert bracelet advising others, including emergency medical staff, of your condition. You must also always carry your EpiPen, and show others how to use it. A few minutes advising others on how to help may save your life.

watch out!

Learn and also teach others to recognize the signs of anaphylaxis. These may differ between sufferers, but any of the following should be taken as an indication that all is not well and emergency treatment needs to be administered:
- metallic taste
- burning or tingling in the mouth
- sudden coughing
- wheezing
- urticaria (hives) on body or face
- tightening of the throat
- swelling of the larynx
- sneezing or running nose
- vomiting
- palpitations
- faintness
- a sense of impending doom

Treating reactions

The best and most effective way to treat a food allergy is to avoid the food completely. This is not always easy. Your problem food may be hidden in among other foods as an ingredient, been prepared alongside or after your trigger food, leaving traces, or you may unwittingly eat something to which you are allergic, for example at a restaurant, a takeaway or at a friend's house.

Product-labelling laws have improved dramatically over the past few years, and many key allergens are now listed on the label. Since November 2005, manufacturers must list the following 12 potential allergens on the label, regardless of quantity: cereals containing gluten, fish, shellfish, eggs, peanuts, nuts, soya, milk and dairy (including lactose), celery, mustard, sesame seeds and sulphites. Also, many supermarkets produce their own 'free from' lists, which are regularly updated. This makes cooking and eating ready meals a much more viable and easy prospect. Over time, living with a food allergy does become easier, as you learn to read labels, to recognize symptoms of a reaction, base your meals around other ingredients, and find alternatives. However, there may always be times when you are caught unaware, and it is important to be prepared to deal with a reaction in any situation.

Medical treatments

Anyone who is severely allergic should carry epinephrine (see page 102) in the form of an EpiPen. You should know how to use it, and educate others in the event of an emergency. You should also be aware of the signs of an impending reaction – the more in tune you are with your body, the quicker you can avert an attack. Your doctor may also prescribe or suggest the following:

Antihistamines

Antihistamines literally block the production of histamine in the body. Histamine is responsible for a large number of symptoms when you suffer

Forms of adrenaline

Adrenaline (epinephrine) can be taken in other forms, apart from the EpiPen, although this is the most often used because it has a long shelf life and is very easy to administer – even someone with no experience can usually get it right. You may however be prescribed one of the following forms:

● Medihaler-Epi. This is normally used if symptoms include swelling of the mouth. This is an aerosol containing adrenaline, and it is normally sprayed directly into the mouth. It is not used when symptoms are more widespread.
● EpiPen. This is very effective in the treatment of severe allergic reactions to foods. It takes the form of an 'auto-injector', and is designed to deliver a single 0.3mg dose of adrenaline into your muscle when where the pen is pushed into your skin. It works with a spring-activated needle. Children who weigh under 25kg are given a 'junior' EpiPen (which delivers 0.15mg); once they exceed 25kg, they are given a larger one.

a reaction to foods. Antihistamines may be used to treat symptoms such as hives, runny nose, itchiness, an irritated throat and abdominal pain associated with an allergic reaction. However, do not make the mistake of believing that a dose in advance of a meal containing the problem food will prevent a reaction. Antihistamines can deal with some symptoms, but by no means all, and they will not avert anaphylaxis. Remember, too, that antihistamines, like all drugs, do have side effects, one of which is often drowsiness (although there are non-drowsy formulas available). They should be used only to quell a reaction, not preventatively, and only on your doctor's instructions.

Antihistamines are sold under a variety of generic and brand names, and are available in both over-the-counter and prescription form. Depending on the type of antihistamine, the drugs can be administered through several different methods, including:

● tablets
● topical creams
● nasal sprays
● eye drops
● liquid

Children and the elderly population should be careful when using antihistamines as among these two groups their side effects can be more pronounced. Potential side effects include drowsiness, irritability and nightmares. Some children may become temporarily hyperactive on antihistamines.

Bronchodilators

If wheezing or symptoms of asthma occur as a result of a food allergy, you will probably be prescribed a bronchodilator which can be inhaled from a handheld pump device, and which can be taken immediately to ease breathing difficulties. Bronchodilators simply work by opening the respiratory passages, relieving symptoms such as shortness of breath or wheezing. They also help to loosen mucus in the lungs, making it easy to expel through coughing. They are usually prescribed in an inhaler form, which allows direct access into the lungs, but they can also be given via tablets, liquids (syrups, usually), or an injection. Bronchodilators can be used either to 'relieve' or 'control' conditions. Long-acting versions will be used to control conditions like asthma, and are normally taken every day as preventatives.

Short-acting bronchodilators are those normally prescribed to food allergy sufferers, and they are only used when there has been a food reaction, or when symptoms appear. Epinephrine (adrenaline) is also a bronchodilator.

Like all drugs, bronchodilators have side effects that may occur in susceptible people. It is recommended that you contact your doctor immediately if you suffer from any of the symptoms listed to the left.

watch out!

There are occasionally serious side effects when taking bronchodilators. You should call your doctor immediately if you experience any of the following symptoms:
- chest pain
- severe headache
- severe vomiting
- fever or chills
- fast or pounding heartbeat
- skin rash
- hives
- hoarseness
- choking or difficulty swallowing
- loud or high-pitched breathing
- worsening of symptoms
- swelling of the face, throat, tongue, lips, eyes, hands, feet, ankles, or lower legs

Corticosteroids (sometimes just called steroids)

These drugs are used to reduce or prevent inflammation (in other words, anti-inflammatory). They are used for a variety of different health conditions. In the case of food allergies, they are used to reduce or prevent inflammation in the respiratory tract, and to relieve or prevent blocked airways. This type of drug is administered through nasal sprays, eye drops, topical creams and injections. Different forms are used for different reasons:

• Corticosteroids by mouth (pills, liquids) and injection can be used to quickly get control over a strong food allergy reaction quickly.

• Some oral corticosteroids are designed for use over several days to control the recurrence of allergy or asthma episodes. They would not generally be used to treat food allergies, but some doctors recommend them.

• Topical corticosteroids may be used to treat itching, swelling, blotching and bouts of eczema that flare up after eating problem foods.

These drugs may be used alongside antihistamines and/or bronchodilators, according to the symptoms that you experience. Corticosteroids can have a wide range of serious side effects, particularly oral forms taken for long periods of time. Inhaled corticosteroids are more localized and do not cause as many side effects. Use them sparingly and only as required.

Self help

Apart from taking whatever medication your doctor or specialist has suggested during a reaction, there are a number of other measures that you can take to help ease symptoms.

• Keep as still as possible when you feel symptoms coming on. If you panic or rush around, your pulse will increase, which can circulate the allergens through your body more quickly.

• If you are suffering from hives, itchiness, facial swelling or blotching, take a series of cool showers, or apply cold compresses, which will help to ease symptoms.

• Lie on your back with your legs elevated if you experience feelings of faintness. This allows the blood to flow to the head, which helps to prevent you from becoming unconscious.

• If symptoms do not ease with your usual medication, or you sense that a serious reaction is at hand, call for an ambulance.

• If it is your first serious reaction, keep a sample of the food (and its wrapping) to take with you to hospital. It's helpful for doctors to work out which food might be causing the problem, and to rule out food poisoning, which can have similar symptoms to food allergy.

Complementary treatments

Apart from taking medication and completely avoiding problem foods, there are other treatments on offer to address food allergies. Some are of limited value, others have been proved successful to some extent, even if on an individual basis; yet more are unfounded and may even be dangerous. These other treatments are often referred to as complementary and alternative medicine (or CAM).

Unfortunately, the success of some complementary systems of medicine has encouraged an industry to build up around them, and there are many unqualified practitioners around who will make promises they cannot keep, and who may even endanger your health. If you do wish to try an alternative therapy or complementary treatment, *always* make sure you choose an experienced practitioner who has been registered with the appropriate regulatory board or body. Experience in dealing with food allergies is also a must, as severe reactions can be life threatening.

The idea behind complementary medicine is that it complements not replaces orthodox medicine. It should be undertaken alongside your normal treatment, and both your doctor and your complementary practitioner should be aware of what the methods are being used or taken to treat or prevent the allergies. Do not stop taking medication prescribed by your doctor unless he gives the all clear; no professional practitioner should ever suggest this.

Having said that, do expect your orthodox medical practitioner to be somewhat sceptical of any complementary treatment you are receiving, and any perceived success. The sciences behind these disciplines are completely different, and there is a fair bit of disdain between camps. You may find your doctor has an open mind, and will take interest in your complementary treatment. In the end, most doctors or practitioners have the same aim – to improve your health and get you well again. Whatever it takes should be acceptable.

Do, however, be wary of practitioners or systems that promise instant results or 'cures'. Chances are that it will take some time for your condition to be stabilized or outgrown, and there is no quick-fix solution to food allergies, no matter what your practitioner tells you. Never undertake a food challenge to anything that has, in the past, caused a serious reaction without a doctor or medical practitioner nearby.

Natural complementary medicine has a fundamentally different approach to health, and you cannot expect to see instant cures or symptomatic relief. Certainly, some treatments will be quick and effective (sometimes within a few minutes of taking a remedy), but longer-term, more chronic conditions will take some time to heal. This does mean adapting your expectations, making long-term health a priority over short-term relief of symptoms. Complementary medicine also works on a preventative basis, building up immunity and energy levels so that you not only overcome whatever allergic condition is troubling you now, but your body will be able to deal with allergies more effectively and efficiently in future.

must know

Choosing a practitioner
This can be difficult. You may wish to consider the following:
• The patient/practitioner relationship is important to the treatment. Choose someone you and/or your child feel comfortable with.
• Ask your doctor if he/she can refer you to a practitioner, or ask friends for practitioners they recommend.
• If you can't find anyone on referral, check with the regulatory board of the therapy you are choosing.
• Check the practitioner's qualifications.
• If you are looking for treatment for your child, make sure the practitioner has experience with children, and is 'child-friendly'.
• Don't be shy about asking for details of what your practitioner thinks he/she can do for you and how.

Homeopathy

Homeopathy is a system of medicine that supports the body's own healing mechanism, using specially prepared remedies. It is 'energy' medicine, in that it works with the body's vital force (natural energy) to encourage healing and to ensure that all body systems are working at optimum level. Homeopathy is often confused with herbalism, partly, perhaps, because some of the remedies are made from herbs. However, herbalists use material concentrations of plants, while homeopathic remedies use plants, minerals and even some animal products as a base. They are prepared through a process known as 'potentization' to bring out their subtle healing properties. We know from modern physics that our seemingly solid bodies are just dense fields of energy. A disturbance in our energy field can give rise to disease, and a potent form of energy can rebalance us. Homeopathy uses 'potentized' remedies to rebalance our body's subtle energy system. Once this is back in balance, the immune system and all the other interconnected systems in our body start functioning better.

The term 'homeopathy' comes from the Greek, meaning 'similar suffering'. It reflects the key principle behind the homeopathic method – that a substance can cure the symptoms in an ill person that it is capable of causing in a healthy person. The idea of using homeopathy for food allergies would be many faceted. Your homeopath would work on the immune system, so that it works more effectively and does not over-react to foods as being foreign substances. You may also be given minute doses of the problem foods 'in potency' (which means that they are diluted to the extent that no traces of the original is present in the remedy, just its 'energy'; this encourages the body to become desensitized.) A homeopath will work on health on all levels, and look at the root causes of your allergy.

Homeopathy and food allergies

It is worth noting that most homeopathic remedies (especially those sold in shops) are made with lactose; if you are lactose-intolerant or suffer from a milk allergy, you may want to avoid these. Hypo-allergenic remedies can be prepared. Reports about whether or not homeopathy works are mixed, but some people have had dramatic success; indeed, a few studies show that it is one of the most effective ways to cure hay fever, which is also an allergic condition. It is entirely safe, as long as you are in the hands of a reputable practitioner, and can easily be practised alongside your normal treatment. Of all the therapies available, this seems the most likely to be effective.

Herbalism

Western herbalism takes a different approach from practitioners trained in the East (China, Japan or India, for example), but it has strong roots in the Western folk tradition, and in much earlier medicine. Herbalism embraces the use of plants, in particular herbs, for healing. Like many other complementary therapies, it is based on a holistic approach to health, and treatment by a practitioner will be undertaken after an assessment of your individual symptoms as well as lifestyle factors and overall health. Like drugs, many herbs have a specific effect on symptoms or a part of the body. The difference is, however, that they are natural and aimed at stimulating your body to return to health by strengthening its systems, as well as attacking the cause of your food allergy itself. Herbs can also be used in much the same way as drugs to address symptoms.

One or many herbs may be administered in different forms, depending on your symptoms and all of the information that you have provided to your herbalist. Herbs can also be used successfully at home, but it's important to remember that they are powerful healing agents and can be toxic in high doses. There are a variety of different forms, including creams, lotions, ointments,

must know

Finding a therapist or therapy
The British Complementary Medicine Association (BCMA) provides a wealth of information about complementary therapies and can put you in touch with a reputable organisation, and give the low-down on hundreds of treatments offered. Call 0845 345 5977 or visit www.bcma.co.uk.
The British Institute for Allergy and Environmental Therapy is a good starting point if you are looking for a registered, approved practitioner or therapy: Ring 01974 241376 or visit www.allergy.org.uk.
The Complementary Medical Association is the largest professional membership body for complementary medical practitioners in the world. The site offers a 'find a practitioner' database, an encyclopaedia of complementary medical therapies, information on specific conditions and a drug/herb/supplement interaction database. Visit www.the-cma.org.uk.

watch out!
Many herbs are not safe for children or people with health conditions, and some can exacerbate allergic reactions or change the effect of any medication you are taking. You must always make sure your practitioner and doctor or specialist are aware of anything you are taking – herbs and drugs alike.

teas, compresses, tinctures (preserved in alcohol), powders, tablets and syrups. They may also be used in the bath to ease symptoms.

Herbalism has received a great deal of scientific interest over the past decade or so, and there have been many studies into the therapeutic use of herbs. One study found that it significantly improved eczema in patients (which is also an allergic condition), and a study from Belgium showed that children with severe asthma improved dramatically with herbal treatment. Given that both of these are conditions related to immune system dysfunction, it cannot hurt to try herbal remedies if you are careful to use a registered, experienced and trained practitioner who is happy for you to continue to use your conventional medication alongside (see page 107).

Acupuncture

Acupuncture balances the body's energy to encourage it to heal itself. Chinese medical practitioners believe that a vital force, called 'chi', flows through our body in channels, or meridians. When this vital force, or energy, becomes blocked or stagnant, disease and disharmony result. Acupuncture works by stimulating or relaxing points along the meridians to unblock energy and to encourage its flow. Thin, solid needles are typically inserted 0.3 to one centimetre ($\frac{1}{10}$ to $\frac{4}{10}$ inch) deep. The acupuncture points are then stimulated either by gentle twirling, heat, or stimulation with a weak electrical current. Occasionally herbs are burnt at acupuncture points and this technique is called moxibustion. Most people feel only a tingling sensation when the needles are inserted; some feel nothing at all. As energy is redirected in the body, chemicals and hormones are stimulated and healing begins to take place.

The World Health Organization recognizes the use of acupuncture in the treatment of a

must know

Acupuncture
Acupuncture is widely and successfully used for a variety of different health conditions; but evidence to suggest that it is successful in the diagnosis and treatment of food allergies is minimal. You may wish to try Nambudripad's Allergy Elimination Technique (NAET), based on the notion that allergies are caused by 'energy blockage' that can be diagnosed with muscle-testing and permanently cured with acupressure and/or acupuncture treatments.

wide range of medical problems, including allergies (although not specifically to food). One study, which looked at the treatment of type one allergic diseases (allergic asthma, rhinitis and urticaria) found that acupuncture had an extensive and 'remarkable' action and worked better than desensitization therapies. Many patients report reduced symptoms and need for medicine after this therapy. And some studies show that people do have lower levels of the allergy-related antibody immunoglobulin E (IgE) in their blood after this therapy. If you can bear the needles, you may have some success.

Nutritional therapies

It makes sense that nutritional therapies should be considered for anyone with food allergies; indeed, many allergy specialists, clinics and doctors provide the services of a nutritionist or dietitian in order to ensure that a balanced diet is maintained despite food restrictions. Some sufferers wish to go one step further and use food and nutritional supplements to encourage better overall health, so that their bodies and immune systems are more effective (and, indeed, work properly!). Many practitioners will help to work on individual health complaints and symptoms, and address specific food allergies and intolerances. This is a safe therapy, but only in the hands of an experienced professional.

Nutritional therapy is a sophisticated system of healthcare, which depends on an increasingly broad-based knowledge of biochemistry, physiology and chemistry to use the tools available within nutrition to address the health needs of the individual. There are three basic diagnoses which are made by the nutritional therapist, and they are allergy (or intolerance), nutritional deficiencies (often sub-clinical, or very minor) and toxic overload.

Nutritional therapists have trained specifically in nutrition. Some may be medical doctors, although this is rare. Specialist medical doctors or consultants will more likely be called medical or clinical nutritionists. The practitioners of other complementary therapies, such as naturopathy, homeopathy and herbalism may also be trained as a nutritional therapist, and offer it as part of the treatment. A wide variety of tests are often used to diagnose deficiencies, and many of these involve 'orthodox' blood testing methods. Be wary of some of the less orthodox methods described in Chapter

Supplements

Never take supplements in high doses unless you have been advised to do so by a registered, experienced nutritional practitioner. Many vitamins, minerals and other substances work in harmony with one another, are toxic in high doses, and will upset your body's biochemistry, and others can affect the medication you may be taking. Most children and adults will benefit from a good all-round multi-vitamin and mineral tablet, with short-term supplementation to clear up deficiencies; however, anything above this must be undertaken with caution and under supervision.

Three. Be wary too of someone who claims to be a nutritionist but is unregistered with the BDA (see page 190) or the Nutrition society (www.nutritionsociety.org).

There is plenty of scope for using nutritional therapy alongside your conventional treatment, as a balanced diet is crucial for overall health and wellbeing. There is also a wealth of evidence suggesting that supplementing vitamins, minerals and other products, such as probiotics, evening primrose oil, and essential fatty acids, can help to treat a wide range of health conditions, including those associated with allergies. For example, several studies showed that asthma and eczema, both allergic conditions linked to food allergies in many cases, have responded well to treatment with fish oils (obviously not appropriate for fish allergy sufferers) and evening primrose oil. Other research indicates that improving overall nutrition, in order to ensure that the immune system is working effectively, and making sure that 'trace' mineral deficiencies are addressed, can make a difference to the severity of symptoms.

Traditional Chinese Medicine

Traditional Chinese Medicine (TCM) is a holistic system of medicine that embraces a wide range of therapies, including herbalism, acupuncture (see page 112), acupressure, diet, massage, exercise (including QiGong) and lifestyle factors. Many people swear by the Chinese approach, which believes that health is not just the absence of symptoms, but the presence of a vital and dynamic state of wellbeing. Many Chinese practitioners are very experienced in dealing with allergic conditions, such as asthma, eczema and food allergies, and can offer treatment to ease symptoms when a reaction takes place. But do be cautious. Chinese herbs in particular are very powerful, and many can be toxic, or even cause damage. Do not take anything without consulting your doctor, and having a clear understanding of potential side effects, and the ingredients contained in any medicines offered.

Ayurveda

Ayurvedic medicine (Indian medicine) is fast gaining acceptance in the West, and as a system of medicine, addressing all aspects of health, it can be a good choice for someone who is struggling due to chronic food allergies. Some of the elements of Ayurvedic medicine include: a type of aromatherapy, breathing, detoxification, diet, exercise, herbs, manipulation of vital energy points (called marma), meditation, music therapy, techniques aimed at emotional and psychological health, yoga and meditation.

The basic Ayurvedic belief is that everything within the universe, including ourselves, is composed of energy or 'prana'. By balancing that energy within, practitioners promote health on all levels. Ayurvedic practitioners believe that we comprise constantly changing energy. Ayurvedic practitioners often work on the immune system, in order to balance its energies and keep it strong so that it is able to fight invaders and relieve chronic conditions. There are seven main constitutional types, and once your child's type is established, he'll be given a set of guidelines to follow, which are an individually prepared plan for health, mind and spiritual maintenance.

Every Ayurvedic programme is completely different and tailored to the individual. There is no one treatment that works for an ailment in every person. The combination of energies in one person might lead to optimum health but in another person, that balance of energies may cause illness. Ayurvedic medicine can, in theory, address any type of health problem, and is particularly useful for shifting long-term or chronic conditions. There is some evidence that food allergies, as well as related conditions such as eczema, hay fever and asthma, have been successfully treated in patients. This treatment is, for the most part, gentle, although the same cautions hold true (see opposite).

Although Ayurveda is mainly a gentle type of medicine that addresses lifestyle rather than just symptoms, it is important to remember that herbs, whatever their source, can be powerful and potentially dangerous to health when administered incorrectly. Similarly, fasting and detoxification techniques may be inappropriate for anyone on a restricted or limited diet due to food allergies.

Staying well

Food allergies do not have to mean the end of healthy, delicious and varied meals, and they certainly do not exclude eating out, or entertaining. While you will definitely have to adapt your lifestyle and eating habits to a greater or smaller degree, and become accustomed to reading labels, asking questions, and working with fewer ingredients when cooking, it really is just a question of becoming accustomed to a new way of life.

Eating out

Whether you are eating out with friends, ordering a takeaway or having a meal in a restaurant, you can eat safely and enjoy many different foods, even if your diet is extremely restricted.

Restaurants and takeaways

One of the biggest causes of reactions when dining out is a fear of asking questions and requesting alternatives. Many people are too shy or embarrassed to discuss their food allergies, particularly when a restaurant is busy and staff seem to be overstretched. But remember, a little courage and some explanation can ensure that you enjoy what should be a normal part of life.

Here are some key tips: do not rely on descriptions of foods. Methods of cooking (for example, in hot oil which has also been used to cook fish or something else to which you might be allergic, or cooking in a pan that is also used to prepare food with sesame oil) should be explained upon request. Not all ingredients are listed in a description; for example, a pizza clearly contains cheese and wheat, but only the toppings will be listed. Ask some questions. And be prepared to ask for details: is there any fish, wheat, milk, sesame or tomato used in the preparation of this meal? Are foods containing these ingredients cooked nearby? If the waiter does not know, ask him to check with the chef.

Avoid the following, which may prove dangerous

• Buffets can be problematic because serving utensils are shared, foods are kept close to one another, and sometimes the food has not been prepared on the spot, so you may not be able to ask the chef what is included.

• Bakeries may also prove difficult, as food is placed close to other foods in display cases, which makes it easier for allergens to spread. Many baked goods are brushed with or include egg, dairy produce and wheat (three of the big allergens) and it is almost impossible to find something that has not been 'tainted' by these ingredients.

• Restaurants that purchase large numbers of dishes or ingredients. Pub meals, smaller restaurants and chains are most likely to be included here. Ask if the food is prepared on the premises, and if it is cooked from 'scratch'. No chef or restaurant owner can ever guarantee food that has been prepared elsewhere. Call in advance if you are unsure.

• If you suffer from peanut, tree nut, sesame, fish or shellfish allergies, you may need to rule out a number of Asian dishes and restaurants. These foods are commonly used in this type of ethnic cooking, and cross-contamination is almost inevitable. That's not to say you can't enjoy a Thai curry or an Indian meal from time to time, but you will need to choose carefully, and ensure that all staff members are aware of your allergy.

• It goes without saying that seafood restaurants are not a good choice for fish or seafood allergy sufferers. The risks are simply too high, even if they can prepare you something off the menu, or without these ingredients.

• Order simple dishes, and ask for sauces and condiments to be served on the side. A plain baked potato with chilli con carne sounds fine if you aren't allergic to any of these things, but you never know what might have been added to the chilli in the process of cooking, or, indeed, how it was cooked. So get your baked potato – a known quantity – and ask for the chilli on the side, so that if you get an early warning symptom, your entire meal won't be ruined. Remember, too, that condiments are notorious for having allergens present. Worcestershire sauce, gravies, hot sauces and even pasta sauces can hide a wealth of different problematic ingredients.

• Don't think you have to rely on a bowl of plain rice or a plate of chips for your meal. Plenty of herbs, spices and other ingredients can be used in the preparation of delicious meals. If you see that the restaurant you have chosen does lovely Italian sauces, ask for 100 per cent durum wheat pasta or sautéed potatoes with olive oil, fresh basil, black pepper and roasted cherry tomatoes. All plain ingredients that mix up to a feast! Do note, however, that some spices may cause a reaction if you are highly atopic (see page 19).

• Go prepared. If you sense the onset of a reaction, don't hesitate to take your emergency medication, and stop eating immediately.

Ask other people with food allergies to recommend a good restaurant. Many are happy to undertake a special request or to cook 'off the menu'. Call in advance if you are concerned. Remember, most restaurant owners would be appalled to discover that someone became ill on their premises. Not only is it not good for business, but it is in their best interest to be able to cater for as many people as possible, and given that food allergies and intolerance are undoubtedly on the increase, you should find that your requirements are catered for.

Entertaining and eating with friends

Most hosts usually ask if there are any foods off the menu before you visit their homes for the first time; but, if they do not, make sure you explain your allergies when you accept an invitation. It is not that difficult to leave out a few ingredients or dishes, and most hosts will be happy to accommodate. If necessary, you can always ask what is on the menu and bring along your own allergen-free version. It is probably not good social etiquette to demand that a separate meal be prepared for you, and many hosts are not accustomed to dealing with food allergies. So if necessary offer some advice ('just use 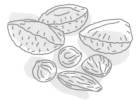 olive oil instead of butter and I can eat it', or 'can you put the nuts in a bowl to be sprinkled rather than adding them to the sauce?') if necessary, and explain that you are perfectly happy to bring along your own food if your allergies do not fit in with the menu planned. Many people will be unaware that using the same spoon to stir the prawns and the rice will cross-contaminate, and that a 'little' of a food allergen might be enough to send a sensitive person into a full-blown reaction. If your allergies are serious and your reactions worrying, you need to make it clear that you can't eat at the table if prawns/nuts/fish are being served. It is easy enough for most hosts to adjust a menu with this knowledge to hand. Once again, don't be shy.

No matter how restrictive your diet, you can also entertain successfully. First of all, remember that just because a particular food is off the menu for you, it doesn't need to affect your guests. Some sufferers are incredibly sensitive and can't even be in the same room as a nut or an egg, but the vast majority can handle foods (using thin surgical gloves if necessary) and prepare healthy meals.

Much of the Western diet is based on dairy produce, eggs, and wheat, and ethnic cuisine tends to use a great deal of sesame and nuts and their oils, as well as seafood and fish. Does that mean you can't prepare these foods? No, it does not. Pizza can, for example, easily be made with alternative flours (see page 121) and soya cheese; similarly, soya or rice milk and a vegan margarine can be used to make a good white sauce. Egg allergy sufferers who are not intolerant to wheat can eat 100 per cent durum wheat and egg-free pastas available at health food shops and supermarkets. Thai, Indonesian or Indian curries can be made successfully using fresh herbs and coconut milk, leaving out the fish sauce and the fish itself. Don't be afraid to experiment. The liberal use of herbs, spices, fresh fruit and vegetables, good-quality meats, soya and soya cheeses and milk, rice milk, and even potatoes and their flour can make adapting a boring dish into something quite wonderful. Bacon, for example, is generally fine for many sufferers, and even those with a sensitivity or allergy to nitrates can choose brands cured without their use; bacon is a good all-round flavour to add to many pasta and rice dishes, and to flavour gravies and sauces. Cook a whole chicken and use the stock to flavour other meals. Use plenty of olive oil, olives and Mediterranean herbs to prepare and to garnish meals. There are plenty of good cookbooks now available for people suffering from food allergies, and even more free recipes on the internet. See page 188 for books and websites to check out.

Allergen free cooking

Substituting non-allergenic ingredients in a recipe is not as hard as you think. Below you'll find some simple tips for adapting favourite recipes, as well as some recipes that cut out most of the main allergenic ingredients without affecting the taste, consistency or success of the recipes.

Egg substitutes

There are several ways in which to substitute an egg in a recipe. For each egg, substitute one of the following:

As *binders*
½ large mashed banana
75ml apple sauce or puréed prunes
1 tbsp ground flaxseed mixed with 3 tbsp water
1½ tbsp water, 1½ tbsp oil, and 1 tsp baking powder
Combine one packet of unflavoured gelatine with one cup boiling water;
**   3 tbsp of this mixture equals one egg**
1 tbsp apricot puree
75ml soft tofu
75ml soy milk

As *leavening*
2 tbsp carbonated water and 2 teaspoons baking flour
1 tsp baking powder, 1 tbsp water, and 1 tbsp vinegar (add vinegar separately at
**   the end for rising)**
Dissolve 1 tsp yeast in ¼ cup warm water
1 heaped tbsp of soy flour and 1 tbsp water
1 tbsp bean flour and 1 tbsp oil
1 tbsp of arrowroot powder mixed with 3 tbsp water
1 tbsp cornstarch mixed with 3 tbsp water
2 tbsp gluten flour or unbleached white flour, 1½ tsp corn oil, ¼ tsp baking
**   powder, and 2 tbsp water**

For *beating*
¼ teaspoon xanthan gum with about ¼ cup of water. Let stand. It thickens, and
**   can be beaten like an egg white.**

Wheat flour substitutes

There are many flours that can be substituted in place of regular flour when baking gluten-free products. This list does not mention them all.

Amaranth flour (made from the seed of the Amaranth plant, which is a leafy vegetable; it is high in protein and very tasty, but it does not stick together well when cooked on its own. Use in combination with other flours, to make cakes and biscuits.

Buckwheat flour should be used in small amounts only because it has a very strong flavour and is sometimes difficult to digest.

Carob flour can be used in cakes, biscuits, drinks, desserts and sweets.

Corn flour can be blended with cornmeal when making breads or muffins.

Nut or legume flours can be used in small portions to enhance the taste of puddings, biscuits, or home-made pasta.

Potato starch flour is excellent for baking when used with other flours. It is a good thickening agent for soups.

Quinoa flour makes excellent biscuits, but it can be quite bitter. You may need to add more sweeteners than usual.

Rice flour is a good thickening agent, and can be blended with other flours for baking.

Soy flour has a nutty flavour and should be used in combination with other flours in baked products that contain nuts, chocolate, or fruit.

Milk substitutes

In most recipes, simply using water or fruit juice is perfectly acceptable. You may also choose to use soya or rice milk.

Cheese and other dairy produce substitutes

In many cases, goat's or ewe's cheese will be fine for cases of intolerance, although not for anyone suffering from milk allergies. Use a soya-based cheese, or omit entirely. Live, organic yoghurt is often acceptable for people suffering from intolerance (see page 156), but if you have a milk allergy, use a soya-based yoghurt instead.

Favourite meals with no fuss

Here are some well-tested recipes that do not contain the majority of food allergens. If you do find an ingredient to which you are sensitive or allergic, you can usually drop it without affecting the taste or consistency of your meal, or move on to something else!

Thai green chicken curry

Serves 4

This is a delicious and largely allergen-free Thai recipe that is both easy to cook and amazingly fragrant. If you aren't allergic to fish, you can substitute a white fish for the chicken, adding it 10 minutes before the end of cooking time.

4 good-sized chicken breasts, skinned, boned and cut into
   chunks
1 tbsp olive oil
2 x 400ml/14fl oz tins coconut milk
1 large mango, peeled and cut into 2-cm (3/4-in.) cubes

For the marinade:
1 stem lemon grass, chopped
Handful of coriander, chopped
1 tbsp olive oil
1 lime, juiced and zest grated

For the curry paste:
2 medium red chillies, halved and de-seeded
1 lime, juiced and zest grated
2 stems lemon grass, roughly chopped
2.5-cm (1-in.) piece fresh root ginger, peeled and sliced
4 cloves garlic, peeled
1 small onion, peeled and quartered

To garnish:
3 level tbsp chopped fresh coriander leaves

Marinate your chicken breasts overnight with a little chopped lemon grass, a handful of coriander, the olive oil and the juice and zest of a lime. Drain the marinade, and fry gently in 1 tbsp olive oil until seared, but not cooked. Put to one side.

Empty the coconut milk into the pan or wok and stir while you bring it up to the boil, then reduce the heat to medium and cook until the fat separates from the solids. This will take 20 minutes or so, and you will have about 570ml (1 pint) left. In some cases, it can be difficult to get the fat to separate, but don't panic. The recipe is just as delicious and works just as well with reduced coconut milk. Meanwhile, make the curry paste: put everything in a food processor or blender and whiz until you have a rather coarse, rough-looking paste.

Now, over a medium heat, add the curry paste and chicken to the pan and, once it has reached simmering point, leave it for about 10 minutes. Finally, add the mango and cook for a further 2 minutes. Sprinkle over the coriander and serve with Thai fragrant rice as an accompaniment. To prepare the curry in advance, follow recipe as above, keeping the paste covered in the fridge, then, 10 minutes before you want to serve, bring the coconut milk back up to the boil, and add the paste, chicken and mango as above. Garnish with fresh coriander and serve.

Gnocchi with sage and lemon sauce

Serves 4

This recipe was supplied by Antoinette Savill (see page 188, Further reading), who has produced a number of fantastic recipes for allergy sufferers. Delicious!

For the gnocchi:
1kg/2lb 4oz floury organic potatoes, peeled and cubed
1 heaped tsp egg replacer substitute (see page 120) and
    2 tbsp cold filtered water
200g/7oz potato flour
85g/3oz vegan margarine
15g/¹/2oz sage leaves, finely chopped
Freshly ground black pepper
Extra potato flour for dusting
1 tsp fine salt

For the sauce:
3 heaped tbsp vegan margarine
1 heaped tbsp dried sage leaves
Rind of 1 unwaxed lemon, freshly grated

To serve:
15g/¹/4oz basil leaves, shredded
Grated pecorino or soya cheese, if tolerated

Boil the potatoes until soft enough to mash, drain them and return them to the pan. Mash the potatoes and then mix in all the gnocchi ingredients and allow to cool. Dust your hands with the extra flour and shape the mixture into walnut-sized pieces, working very lightly. When they are the correct size, press the back of a fork a little way into the gnocchi to decorate with the traditional ridges.

Bring a large pan of water to the boil with a teaspoon of salt, and drop the gnocchi into the boiling water in batches, but make sure that you keep them apart. Cook them for about a minute, or until they float to the top. Lift them out with a slotted spoon and place in a warmed bowl; this way you can keep them warm while cooking the rest of the batches in the same way.

In a small saucepan, melt the margarine, with the sage leaves, in a small saucepan until bubbling, then remove from the heat. Sir in the grated lemon and drizzle the sauce over the gnocchi. Serve with shredded basil leaves, plenty of black pepper, and accompany with a bowl of grated cheese.

Sweet potato, chickpea and parsley mash

Serves 1-2
Also one of Antoinette's recipes (see page 188, Further reading), this makes a great side dish – or even a meal for youngsters.

**1 large organic sweet potato, peeled, chopped and steamed until
    soft**
2 heaped tbsp chickpeas, cooked without salt or sugar
100ml/3½fl oz water
1 tbsp fresh parsley
Salt and freshly ground black pepper
2 tsp olive oil

To serve:
Chopped parsley

Put the cooked potato into a food processor, blend briefly until it becomes a lumpy mash and then add the chickpeas and water. Process until a coarse mash is achieved and stir in the parsley. Season to taste and drizzle with good-quality olive oil and a little fresh parsley to serve.

Chocolate soda bread

Serves 6–8

This recipe was supplied by Antoinette Savill (see
page 188, Further reading), who has produced a
number of recipes for allergy sufferers.

450g/1lb gluten-free white flour mix, plus some for
    dusting
2 tsp unrefined caster sugar
1 tsp salt
2 tsp gluten-free bicarbonate of soda
100g/3½oz dairy and nut-free chocolate (dark
    chocolate; check the label), roughly chopped
400ml/14fl oz buttermilk (often OK for milk allergy
    sufferers, but when in doubt, use rice or soya
    milk instead)

Preheat the oven to 200°C/400°F/Gas 6. Sieve the
flour, sugar, salt and bicarbonate of soda into a
bowl, mix together and then stir in the chocolate.
Make a well in the centre of the mixture and pour
in the buttermilk. Using clean hands, bring the
mixture together into a soft but not wet and sticky
dough. Add a little more 'milk' if necessary to hold
it together. Transfer the dough to a clean board
dusted with some gluten-free flour. Knead lightly
for a few seconds.

Place the dough on a non-stick baking tray and
pat into a thick round about 5-cm/2-in. deep.
Using a sharp knife, score deep markings for six to
eight portions and bake in the oven for about 25
minutes, until bread is cooked through. Serve the
bread when it is just warm.

Easy tricks for family favourites

Basic beef or lamb: Brown 1kg (2¼lb) minced beef (or lamb) in a little olive oil with one diced onion, and add two bay leaves, a grated carrot, a handful of chopped celery, and some fresh basil (a handful of chopped basil leaves is about right), and 250ml/9fl oz vegan stock. Leave to simmer for 20 minutes. You now have the makings of a few different meals. For **shepherd's pie**, allow the mince to dry out a little; as the juices evaporate, add a handful of frozen or fresh peas. Cook for three minutes and, if not allergic, add a little Worcestershire sauce or tomato purée. Season with salt and freshly ground pepper. Stir and put into an ovenproof dish. Parboil two large sweet potatoes (or large white potatoes) for eight minutes, and slice when cool. Place the potato slices on top of the mince, drizzle with olive oil, bake for 30 minutes and serve. For **Bolognese sauce**, use your basic mince recipe, but add a little red wine (if not allergic) and allow the alcohol to burn off (about four minutes). Tomato paste can be added if required. Serve with allergen-free spaghetti or pasta. Or try homemade **hamburgers**: plain mince mixed with salt, pepper, some mixed dried herbs and a smattering of tomato paste. Shape and chill for a couple of hours, and then grill, fry or barbeque. Serve with sweet potato chips, fresh cucumber and tomato relish, on a wheat-free bun.

Chicken ideas: Chicken 'nuggets' or goujons can by made by dipping chicken pieces in a little rice or soya milk, and coating in seasoned potato flour or ground quinoa. Shallow fry or brush with olive oil and grill. Thai, Indian and Moroccan recipes can all be adapted for allergies, so don't hesitate to experiment. Anything is possible as long as you avoid shop-prepared sauces and pastes, and use fresh, whole ingredients.

Italian: Pizza bases and pastas are now readily available in non-allergenic forms. If tomatoes are a problem, roast red peppers and purée with garlic, onions and plenty of fresh basil for an easy sauce to use on pizza or pasta. Use soya yoghurt instead of bechamel sauces, and add a little feta (sheep's milk cheese) or soya cheese for flavour. Even pesto is possible: if you can tolerate goat's or sheep's cheese, use pecorino instead of Parmesan, and blend with olive oil, plenty of fresh basil, and a little garlic for an easy sauce. Pine nuts are low allergen foods, and can normally be toasted and added to the paste without causing problems.

5 Allergic children

Food allergies in children are relatively rare, although studies indicate the incidence is increasing. In the Western world, roughly eight per cent of babies under one month are affected, three per cent of children under the age of five, and less than one per cent of adults. Food intolerance is more common, affecting babies, children and adults – perhaps up to ten per cent or more. The good news is that with a healthy balanced diet, careful weaning, complete avoidance of problem foods, and a sound understanding of emergency treatment, allergic babies and children will not only thrive, but also possibly outgrow their allergies by the time they start school.

Why are children more allergic?

First of all, children of allergic parents are much more likely to suffer from allergies themselves; allergies in this sense also include suffering from asthma, eczema, hay fever and food allergies. Given that allergies do appear to be on the increase in adults, it is not surprising that more and more children are suffering.

Allergies are also most likely to affect babies and young children because of their underdeveloped immune systems. They may have been sensitized to certain foods that their mother ate in the last trimester of pregnancy (see pages 177-78), or they can equally be sensitized by foods that come through their mother's breast milk. In terms of intolerance, children are more vulnerable because they consume, dose for weight, higher doses of food chemicals than adults do. Moreover, many children's diets are not varied, they are weaned too early, they are not breastfed, and problematic foods are introduced to the diet when a child's system is simply unable to cope.

must know

Caesarean babies

Children born by caesarean section are four times more likely to develop proven egg allergies than are children born vaginally, according to a 2003 study. Parents of these children were more than seven times more likely to report the children developing allergies to egg, fish, or nuts. C-section delays the colonization of the baby's gut with beneficial bacteria, which is normally picked up in the birth canal. Also, many women who have caesareans are given antibiotics to prevent infection after surgery, and spend time in hospital which puts a new baby in contact with higher levels of unhealthy bacteria.

Common allergies

In children, the pattern of allergens is different than it is with adults. The most common food allergens that cause problems in children are eggs, milk, peanuts, soya and wheat. Adults usually do not lose their allergies, but children can often outgrow them. Children are more likely to outgrow allergies to milk or soya than allergies to peanuts, fish or shellfish; however, some children outgrow them all. The foods that children react to tend to be foods they eat most often. For example, rice is considered 'low allergen' here, whereas rice allergy in Japan is much more common. Peanut and corn allergies are highest in the US, because these foods and their by-products are used regularly in manufacturing, and eaten regularly. Fish allergies are more common in Scandinavia; shellfish allergies more common in Europe, and in the UK, milk and eggs top the list of offenders.

Symptoms of allergy in kids

One of the main problems in diagnosing a food allergy in children is that they are largely unable to articulate how they are feeling, and do not relate what they eat to the symptoms they experience. For that reason, parents need to be very observant of any change in behaviour, skin, bowel movements, sleep patterns and any other anomaly in the way their children react to a food.

If you or your partner is allergic, there is an increased chance that your child will be too, (between 20 and 40 per cent) so keeping an eye out for symptoms is even more important. If both parents are allergic then this risk is even higher (between 40 and 60 per cent). Food reactions in children can be dramatic, affecting breathing, causing instant swelling, and producing vomiting, but they can also be a little slower to manifest themselves. For this reason, keeping a food diary for your child is very important.

If you are breastfeeding a baby who has symptoms of allergy or intolerance (see panel overleaf), you will need to keep a food diary relating to what *you* eat and the impact (if any) it has on your child. If your baby has eczema, for example, try to work out when the attacks are worse; if her skin becomes itchy after feeds, consider what you have just eaten. You may need to attempt a simple elimination diet, cutting out the key problematic foods, such as cow's milk (and all dairy produce), eggs and wheat to see if that has any impact. After a couple of weeks, introduce them one by one to see if there is any reaction. Be careful, however, not to streamline your diet too much; nursing mothers need plenty of good, healthy food in order to produce good-quality milk.

For toddlers and pre-school children who can't explain how they are feeling, note any symptoms in your food diary, including hyperactive behaviour, sleep problems, wheeziness, irritability, unusual bowel movements (such as particularly smelly or liquid nappies), and anything else unusual. Remember that not all reactions will be instant; some may take up to 48 hours to manifest themselves.

It is important to establish whether food allergies or intolerance are causing symptoms; children with undiagnosed allergies may suffer problems with growth, development, learning, hearing, concentration, sleep and overall wellbeing.

Common symptoms in children

Babies
Crying
Colic
Vomiting
Diarrhoea
Rashes
Urticaria (hives)
Eczema
Cold-like respiratory symptoms
Sleep disturbances
Some babies become seriously ill and fail to thrive

Toddlers and older children
Chronic congestion (and of the nose)
Cheek and ear flushing
Recurrent ear infections and tonsillitis
Sleep disturbances
Abdominal pain
Diarrhoea
Vomiting
Skin rashes (particularly around the mouth)
Urticaria (hives)
Hyperactivity
Temper tantrums
Fatigue
Lymph node swelling
Discolouration around both eyes (almost like black eyes)
Sniffing and snuffling
Wheezing
Shortness of breath
Coughing
Congested ears, affecting hearing

Cow's milk

We looked at the spectrum of cow's milk allergy in Chapter Two of this book. Although adults can be affected by this allergy, it does tend to be children who are most likely to suffer, and the ramifications can be much more dangerous. First of all, for the first six to 12 months of life, milk forms the basis of most babies' diets. If they are unable to tolerate their main source of nutrition and sustenance, it can have a dramatic impact on growth, development and health. Secondly, it is much harder to replace the important nutritional elements of infant formula, breast milk and even cow's milk with other foods or drinks. Up until the age of 12 months, most babies do not have a particularly varied diet, and even toddlers tend to turn their noses up at all-important fruit and vegetables, making it even more difficult to achieve a balanced diet. Relying on supplements is never the answer, and a lack of suitable nutrition can, in some cases, be life threatening.

The problem with cow's milk

Two different elements of cow's milk cause problems – lactose (milk sugar) and milk protein. Each of these substances produces its own particular problems. Lactose is the sugar in milk, and anyone who is intolerant to lactose (see page 25), is likely to be deficient in lactase, the enzyme that helps the body to digest lactose. It is worth noting, however, that lactose occurs in any kind of milk (including breast milk) to some degree. Even in ethnic groups who are more likely to suffer from lactose intolerance (Asians, Africans, native populations from Australia, Canada and America, for example), this condition rarely manifests itself until after three years of age – largely because it would make breastfeeding impossible. The vast majority of healthy, full-term babies can make lactase, which enables them to digest sugar in milk; sometimes premature babies are lactose-intolerant until they reach their original due dates.

Interestingly, too, healthy full-term babies can temporarily become lactose intolerant during and after a bout of diarrhoea, which can cause them to lose the enzyme. They regain their tolerance after the diarrhoea has ended and their bodies have had time to make more of the enzyme.

However, in some populations (some experts put the figure at 80 per cent of all of the world's people; see page 24), as the babies mature their bodies gradually make less and less lactase. As they grow into toddlerhood, they no longer tolerate milk of any kind.

A true milk allergy, rather than an intolerance to lactose, is caused by milk protein. Unlike lactose intolerance, which tends to appear later in toddlerhood or childhood, allergy or intolerance to cow's milk protein is not uncommon in babies, but becomes less common as they grow up. Between two and seven and a half per cent of healthy babies have a significant intolerance to the protein in cow's milk. Children who are born to allergic parents are the most likely candidates. Babies with this type of allergy can experience a wide range of symptoms, from vomiting (when given a cow's milk formula), diarrhoea, colic, abdominal discomfort to rashes, eczema, and consistent crying and even failure to thrive. Even breastfed babies can experience discomfort, as the protein from milk can be passed through breast milk and into the baby's digestive system. That is not to say that breast milk should be ruled out; far from it. It is still the best and most easily digestible form of nutrition for all infants. However, it is essential that the mother of an allergic baby excludes all forms of cow's milk from her diet for the duration of breastfeeding.

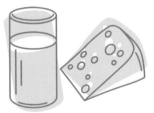

must know

Feeding baby
Lactose intolerance in babies usually manifests itself obviously, with clear discomfort after every feed. Lactose-free cow's milk (or goat's milk) formulas may be tolerated, as should soya-based formulas. Hydrolyzed formulas (see page 137) also work well, although these can be expensive and possibly unnecessary. Breast milk should, however, be the milk of choice for lactose-intolerant babies; lactose rarely crosses into breast milk.

Which milk?

Breast milk is designed to provide complete nourishment for a baby for several months after its birth. Before milk is produced the mother's breast produces colostrum, a deep-yellow liquid containing high levels of protein and antibodies. A newborn baby who feeds on colostrum in the first few days of life is better able to resist the bacteria and viruses that cause illness. This is relevant for several reasons. First of all, when a baby is protected to some degree from potential illness, his immune system will not be under pressure, and will, therefore, be less likely to react in abnormal ways to food and other potential allergens. Secondly, because proteins are implicated in so many food allergies and intolerance cases, it is important that babies receive the most natural and digestible form, which is found in human milk.

The fat contained in human milk, compared with cow's milk, is also more digestible for babies and allows for a greater absorption of fat-soluble vitamins into the bloodstream from the baby's intestine. Food allergies and intolerance are linked to deficiencies of a number of key nutrients – in particular, essential fatty acids (EFAs), which are present in human milk, but not in most infant formulas.

Antigens in cow's milk can cause allergic reactions in a newborn baby, whereas such reactions to human milk are rare. Furthermore, other research has shown that breastfeeding for the first 15 weeks protects against diarrhoeal diseases. This is significant from the point of view that gut dysfunction appears to be related to food intolerance and sensitivity.

It is worth noting that food molecules are also transmitted via breast milk, which makes the breastfeeding mother's diet all important in the fight against allergies. If you are breastfeeding, you must ensure that you eat any potential allergens in moderation, particularly if there are allergies in the family, and try to eat as varied a diet as possible. Not only will your baby have a greater chance of getting the nutrients he needs, but you will also guarantee that he is not in contact with any one potentially allergenic food in high levels.

In Chapter Seven we will look at precautions while breastfeeding in much more detail.

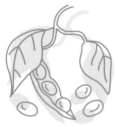

Formula milk

If you can't breastfeed, it is important to choose your
baby's formula with great care. Everything on the market
will be safe, with balanced nutrients and added vitamins,
but you will need to choose between brands according to
your baby's age and special requirements. Most formulas
are based on cow's milk, but there are soya-based
formulas available for babies who have difficulty in
digesting cow's milk, or who have allergies or intolerance.
These, too, may cause problems (see opposite). Children
with a milk-protein allergy may have to switch to a
hydrolyzed or elemental formula (see below). Babies or
toddlers who are lactose-intolerant can be offered a
lactose-free formula, which uses other sugars in the place
of milk sugar.

Soya milk

Soya milk and other soya products have been put forward
as the answer to food allergies and sensitivities. There
are, however, many differing views on this approach, and
it is worth taking them into consideration when adding
soya to your child's diet. Children who are allergic to
cow's milk are, in a high percentage of cases, also at risk
of developing a soya allergy. Soya milk is also not naturally
high in calcium, which children need for many aspects of
growth, including the development of strong teeth and
bones. Most soya formulas contain the recommended
levels of calcium and other nutrients, but some are better
than others. Look out for fortified varieties.

Soya is a food product that has been heavily involved
in genetic modification. Ensure that any soya product
you purchase is GM-free, and preferably organic. Soya is
a prime source of 'phyto-oestrogens', which are natural
compounds that act as weak oestrogens (basically

female hormones). While the phyto-oestrogens have been shown to have a dramatic effect on health in adults (they may offer some protection against conditions such as breast, bowel, prostate and other cancers, cardio-vascular disease and menopausal symptoms), there are concerns over what their long-term effects of phyto-oestrogens may be when given to infants and young children, largely because they can play havoc with hormonal activity.

Hydrolyzed formulas

Also called 'elemental formula', hydrolyzed 'milks' are produced by the heating or 'enzymatic hydrolysis' of cow's milk protein, rendering them hypoallergenic.

If exclusive breastfeeding cannot be established or maintained then a partially hydrolyzed infant milk formula or an extensively hydrolyzed formula is the next best thing. Partially hydrolyzed formulas are not hypoallergenic – don't use one if your baby has a protein allergy (or if you suspect he may have one). However, partially hydrolyzed whey formulas have been shown in one study to reduce atopic dermatitis compared to standard cow's milk formula.

Extensively hydrolyzed formulas are those in which the casein has been extensively broken down combined with additional amino acids, which are the building blocks of protein. These formulas are considered hypoallergenic and are used for babies who have a protein allergy. So, the more complete the hydrolysis process the less allergenic the milk. But extensively hydrolyzed formulas are very expensive and tend to have an unpleasant taste, which is poorly tolerated by older infants. Indeed, unless you get your baby on to this type of formula before about eight weeks of age, you are unlikely to make a successful switch, as the taste is so pronounced.

must know

Goat's milk

Goat's milk is also not usually a good alternative, especially if your child has a problem digesting milk proteins. Goat's milk is low in vitamin D and it is also low in iron, vitamin B12 and folate, which can lead to an iron deficiency or megaloblastic anaemia (low blood counts). If you are going to feed your baby goat's milk, make sure that you use a commercially prepared pasteurized form that is supplemented with vitamin D and folic acid. Like hydrolyzed formulas, goat's milk formulas tend to have a strong, unpleasant taste, and it may take some time for your baby to become accustomed to it. Babies who are lactose-intolerant do not usually have a problem with goat's milk formula.

Weaning

The stage at which you choose to wean your baby will also have an impact on their susceptibility to allergies. Research very clearly shows that leaving first foods as late as possible will help to ensure that your child's digestive system is mature enough to cope.

Six months is a good time to start with a little table food – some rice, a few fruits and vegetables, for example, but leave it longer if you can, particularly if there are allergies of any nature in your family. By seven months your baby should be ready. Don't be tempted to replace the milk in your baby's diet. Until your baby is about a year old, she will get most of her nutrition from her milk. Other foods will add a little variety, and introduce her to new tastes, but they should not be relied upon as a source of a balanced diet. Early foods merely supplement milk feeds, and there is no reason to worry if your baby has nothing but milk for the first six or seven months of life.

Some babies will thrive on milk for the first 12 months, so don't panic if you have a slow beginner. If you wish to stop breastfeeding, you can switch to the bottle long before you need to give solid foods. Similarly, it is not advised that you give solid foods to a baby that is younger than four months old, under any circumstances. It is now believed that a baby's digestive system is not mature enough to cope with solids before this time, and he will be more prone to food allergies, rashes and digestive upsets.

The cautious approach has been proved through a variety of different studies to help prevent allergies and intolerance in susceptible children. For example, one study followed 165 children from birth to age seven years old who were at high risk of developing allergies because of their parents' allergic conditions. Dr Robert S Zeiger, author of the study, concluded: 'Avoiding the early introduction of potentially allergenic foods is the basic step in the primary prevention of food allergies in children who are at high risk, but some infants may still become sensitized or allergic to a food ... fortunately, early detection of a food allergy can help reduce its severity.'

Foods least likely to cause allergic reactions should be introduced first. These include rice and rice cereals (although watch

What foods?

There are certain foods that should not be introduced too early in any child's diet – whether or not there are allergies in the family. Try to stick to these basic guidelines:

• First foods should be introduced one at a time, and any reactions noted (see pages 183-84).
• A recent EU directive lists 12 foods or additives as being the source of the majority of adverse food reactions: these are peanuts, tree nuts, sesame seed, mustard seed, cow's milk, eggs, fish, shellfish, soya, wheat, celery and sulphites. From the age of six months, some of these foods can be introduced one at a time, starting with a small amount and introducing no more than one allergenic food at a time. This group of foods will include wheat, well-cooked egg, cow's milk, fish, shellfish and soya. By the age of 12 months, the majority of high-risk foods should have been introduced (apart from peanuts). However, these guidelines are not appropriate for babies who already have a suspect or proven food allergy, or any other allergic disorder such as asthma or eczema. In such cases, high-allergen foods should be left as late as possible, and introduced upon the advice of a registered dietitian and/or allergy specialist.
• Try to stick to the following time frame: chicken at six months, egg at one year, fish at ten months, chocolate at one year, wheat at nine months, oranges at one year and peanuts and other nuts at three years. These are the most common allergens. If you have an allergic child, hold off as long as possible. Bony fish should not, for example, be offered until at least the age of three.
• Test out beef and chicken cautiously, as these can cross-react with milk and egg allergies respectively. If they seem to cause no problems, include them in your child's diet.
• Shellfish and strawberries can be introduced after your child's second birthday.
• No food should be eaten in large quantities and it is a good idea to avoid giving any one food every day. This does mean being imaginative with your child's diet, but if you try to eat a varied diet as a family, it should be easier to achieve. Try out fruits, vegetables and grains that you may not normally consider buying: sweet potatoes, kale, pulses (such as lentils, black beans), dried unsulphured fruits soaked and puréed, millet, rice, parsnips, kiwi fruit, mango, quinoa, chickpeas and barley.

must know
A balanced diet

It is possible to create a healthy diet around even the most limited number of acceptable foods. Rice dishes, stir-fries, soups, casseroles and stews can all be made using less allergenic foods, and the minimum of seasoning. There are also a number of nutritious snacks which can help to create a balanced diet. These include: oatcakes, rice cakes, grapes, berries, raisins, corn snacks for children, bananas, fruit smoothies, apples, lightly cooked carrots, peppers, mango, frozen pure juice 'lollies', unsugared, gluten-free cereals, fruit bars and even the occasional 'hypoallergenic' (free from those foods to which your child is allergic) biscuit or (if tolerated) soya cheese or soya yoghurt. These make excellent, nutritious snacks, which can help to created a balanced diet.

out for added milk), pear, apple, carrots and potatoes. Other good first foods, include peaches, apricots, bananas (and it is worth noting that very ripe bananas improve the health of the gut, which can be crucial for those susceptible to food allergies), parsnips, swede, green beans, squash, sweet potato, cauliflower and broccoli. Introduce them separately, about a week apart, and keep the diet as varied as possible. The panel opposite will give you some idea of the most and least 'allergenic' foods. Choose from the second list first, moving on to the first only if your child has successfully tolerated most other foods, and is older than a year or so.

Commercially-prepared baby foods are acceptable for allergic babies, but only if: they are prepared in conditions where other allergens (such as peanuts, sesame, milk or wheat) have not been used; they contain only those foods to which your baby has already been successfully introduced; they contain only the ingredients that *should* be there (in other words, in puréed pears, only pear should be present; in mixed vegetables, only vegetables); they have no additives or preservatives and are organic. Additives and preservatives may cause a reaction in some children, which has nothing to do with a true food allergy; also organic foods are less likely to contain chemicals used in farming and production, which may cause reactions. Watch out, however, for the addition of starches and thickeners added to baby foods – and a lot of water, which makes the actual content of food and nutrients much lower.

Which starter food?

Most allergenic foods	Least allergenic foods
berries	apples
buckwheat	apricots
chocolate	asparagus
citrus fruits	avocados
coconut	barley
corn	beetroot
dairy products	broccoli
egg whites	carrots
mustard	cauliflower
nuts	chicken
peas	cranberries
peanut butter	dates
pork	grapes
shellfish	honey
soya	lamb
tomatoes	lettuce
wheat	mangoes
yeast	oats
	papayas
	peaches
	pears
	raisins
	rice
	salmon
	squash
	sweet potatoes
	turkey
	veal

Remember, however, that any food can cause an allergic reaction in a susceptible child, so take care to introduce anything new one at a time, and gauge any reaction before moving on to the next. Avoid mixed and combined foods for as long as possible, unless they contain only foods that have already been successfully introduced.

Eliminating foods

Despite your best efforts, it may become clear that your child has developed an allergy to something in his diet. When weaning is complete, and your child is eating a variety of foods, it can be difficult to work out what the culprit might be.

Using a food diary (see page 72) to record foods and symptoms, including behavioural changes, is your first step (see page 131), but if you find that there is nothing obvious, you can try a very, very basic elimination diet. Under no circumstances should you try the type of elimination diet suggested for adults, as children need a wide variety of foods on a daily basis. You should consult a doctor or allergy specialist before embarking on any elimination programme; however, if your child is still drinking an appropriate formula and/or breastfeeding, you can safely remove a few items without losing the balance. Remember that for the first year of life, babies will get the majority of their nutrition from their usual milk. Many doctors suggest that allergic babies stay on this milk for the first two years of life, to ensure that all nutrient needs are met. For two to three weeks, stick to the foods suggested below, and then gradually introduce his normal foods to the diet, one by one again, leaving the most problematic foods (eggs, milk, wheat, fish, shellfish, nuts, sesame) until last.

Under six months:
You can usually return to formula or breast milk only; although if your baby has been taking a cow's milk formula, you will probably need to change to one that is hydrolyzed.

Six months to two years:
Hydrolyzed formula or breast milk (although, in the latter case, you will need to cut out potential allergens from your diet at the same time, see page 141).
Rice cereal and rice cakes
Lamb or chicken
Cooked pears or bananas

Over two years:
Rice cereals, rice, rice cakes and rice bread
Lamb and chicken
Cooked or canned pears, apricots, prunes or their juices
Sunflower or olive oil, vegan, allergen-free margarine
Cooked beetroot, sweet potato, carrots, parsnips
Lettuce

Some experts recommend that you offer a good vitamin and mineral supplement alongside, which contains iron and calcium. A good one to try, in syrup form, is Forceval. Another acceptable alternative for the older age group is to offer dried, unsulphered apricots and prunes (for their iron content) as well as calcium-enriched rice milk.

This diet is not supremely well balanced, but it provides adequate nutrition for a short period of time. Under no circumstances should it be continued for longer than three weeks. If you can not find the culprit even after reintroducing all your child's usual foods, allergy testing (see page 77) will probably be required, and can be arranged by your doctor. Babies under the age of one will not normally be tested, so try to stick to a hypoallergenic diet as much as possible – and incorporate the same elements into your own diet if you are breastfeeding.

Another alternative

The other way to use elimination is to remove foods, one by one, for a week or so, to see if symptoms clear up. The obvious place to start is by removing the key allergenic foods. But remember, it can take a couple of weeks for food to completely clear the body completely, so short-term avoidance of a food may not have a dramatic effect on symptoms. In the case of true allergy, symptoms should resolve more quickly than in the case of intolerance. Always take steps to replace the nutrients found in any food you are choosing to eliminate. For example, if you cut out dairy, increase calcium-rich foods. Only eliminate one food at a time. This may be time-consuming, but it will prevent an imbalance in the diet.

Other nasties

You may be frustrated to find that you can't pinpoint your child's allergy or intolerance, and have equally frustrating results with conventional allergy tests. There may, however, be another cause. Many children (and indeed adults) are sensitive to food additives (in Europe, known as 'E-numbers'), nitrates and other things added or occurring naturally in foods, such as salicylates.

Food additives

Food processing has increased a great deal over the past couple of decades, and there are now literally hundreds of additives used regularly in the making of children's food. Many experts believe that these chemicals place an extra strain on immature systems, making children that much more susceptible in the present and perhaps laying down the foundation for allergies in the future. Food additives have only rarely been shown to cause true allergic (immunological) reactions; however, they can cause reactions and symptoms much like intolerance in sensitive kids.

Monosodium glutamate (MSG)

Monosodium glutamate (MSG) is a food additive that enhances flavour by stimulating the taste buds. After MSG was linked to brain damage in infant laboratory animals in 1970, manufacturers agreed to stop adding it to baby food. But MSG is still commonly added to many products, including tinned soup, convenience foods, flavoured crisps, fried chicken batter and Chinese food. Foods that are chemically close enough to MSG, and thought to produce similar reactions, include hydrolyzed vegetable protein and yeast extract.

Symptoms of MSG sensitivity include: dizziness, nausea, skin rash, migraine headache, asthma-type symptoms, flushing and tremors.

Sulphites

Sulphites are another problem. They are sometimes used to preserve the colour of foods such as dried fruits and vegetables, and to inhibit the growth of micro-organisms in fermented foods such as wine. Sulphites are safe for most people. A small segment of the population, however, has been found to develop shortness of breath or fatal shock shortly after exposure to these preservatives. Sulphites are capable of producing severe asthma attacks in sulphite-sensitive asthmatics (see page 60).

Food colours

Reactions to food colours tartrazine (E 102, a yellow food colour) and carmine (E 120 or red cochineal) have been reported occasionally in sensitive individuals. Symptoms include skin rashes, nasal congestion and hives, although the incidence is very low. IgE-mediated allergic reactions have been reported for carmine. Tartrazine has also been reported to cause asthma in sensitive individuals.

Salicylates

Salicylates, another problem, are found naturally in many fruits and vegetables and are added to some food products. Foods naturally high in salicylates include berries, grapes, oranges, dried fruit, olives, tomatoes, tea, some herbs and spices, as well as some liquorice, peppermint, and honey products. Some people are sensitive to salicylates and can only handle small quantities. This sensitivity can be manifested in many ways including headaches, lack of concentration, cognitive and perceptual disorders, breathing problems, and hyperactivity.

Not only are food additives a major cause of health problems, but they can play havoc with an immature system, affecting growth, mood, concentration, sleeping patterns and overall resistance to infection by overloading a child's system with toxins. Children's food is full of some of the worst additives, largely because manufacturers (rightly) believe that something brightly coloured, over-sweetened, and refined and processed to look like your child's favourite cartoon character is more likely to appeal to a faddy child. As boring as it may sound, learn to read the labels, and take some time to educate yourself about this problem. Choosing, fresh, natural ingredients and avoiding processed food of any description is the very easiest way to ensure that your child is not in contact with potential allergens.

Hyperactivity

Hyperactivity is a descriptive term that refers to restless, distractible children who have poor impulse control, often display abrupt mood swings, have inappropriate anger, and are sometimes violent. Their schoolwork suffers from inattention, disorganization, and poor memory, and their behaviour is disruptive.

Hyperactive behaviour and a lack of concentration are often connected and so the term attention deficit hyperactivity disorder (ADHD) was coined. The current conventional treatment is to offer medication, in particular Ritalin, which has the effect of calming children. There is an increasing wealth of evidence, however, to suggest that it is the Western diet, food allergies and intolerance, and an overall lack of exercise that may actually be at the root of the problem.

There has been some interesting research. For example one study found that 74 per cent of 261 hyperactive kids tested had problems with sugar consumption, in that it affected their mood and energy levels much more dramatically than in other children. In another study, which offered 76 children a low-allergen diet, 62 improved and 21 achieved completely normal behaviour. Other symptoms such as headaches and fits improved. The worrying thing is that up to 48 foods were incriminated, with artificial colourings and preservatives being the worst culprits!

Suspect foods include all forms of refined sugar and any products that contain it, artificial colours,

did you know?

In one small study, the hyperactivity ratings of 19 out of 26 children given a diet excluding wheat, corn, yeast, soya, citrus, egg, chocolate, peanuts and artificial colours and flavours, dropped from an average of 25 (high) to an average of eight (low).

flavourings or preservatives, and foods that contain salicylates (including almonds, apples, apricots, cherries, currants, all berries, peaches, plums, prunes, tomatoes, cucumbers and oranges). Food allergies may also cause symptoms of hyperactivity, so start to keep a food diary to see if you can pinpoint what the problem might be. An elimination diet (see page 142) will help if you can not find the cause.

Several studies show that many children with ADHD will have symptoms and signs of delayed pattern food allergy – which is very difficult to detect through testing, as reactions appear far too late. The most common symptoms are allergic shiners (dark circles under the eyes) and stuffy nose. ADHD kids tend to have histories of nose congestion, recurrent middle-ear infections, and sleep disturbances, starting in infancy. Some have more specific allergic problems such as eczema, hives, and asthma but most have non-specific symptoms that do not fit the familiar patterns of allergy. Digestive disturbances are common but may occur only infrequently; some children have bouts of diarrhoea while others tend to be constipated. Some have headaches and many have leg pains, often at night.

If these symptoms fit your child, it would be well worth considering an overhaul of his diet with the help of a nutritionist/dietitian or allergy specialist. It would mean cutting out on refined foods of all descriptions, lowering sugar intake, removing additives, preservatives, and foods containing salicylates, and work on eliminating the most common food allergens, one by one.

Being prepared

Whether your child's allergies are dramatic, with life-threatening reactions, or lower-key, with more niggling health complaints, it is extremely important to adopt a healthy eating plan, cutting out all offending foods and replacing them with nutritious alternatives.

Do not be overwhelmed by the prospect of an allergic child, no matter how serious the reactions; with common sense, adept label-reading, a handful of good recipes, and a carefully put together action plan for emergencies, life can pretty much return to normal. Indeed, kids with allergies, even on strict diets, are often extremely healthy, as the 'junk' fare that so many kids of today live on are almost always excluded from their diets.

Children can be taught to understand their health problems, but chances are they will feel isolated and 'different' when their diets are unlike those of their friends, and the daily fare and treats that punctuate the life of an average child simply do not exist. Fortunately, there are a wealth of child-friendly recipes and recipe books now available to help you prepare foods that are pretty much the norm in any age group.

It can also help to involve your child in the selection, preparation and cooking of food from an early age – not only will he be given some choice in what he eats, which can be greatly empowering within a limited diet, but he can also learn to try things he may not otherwise have considered. What is more, you don't want a child growing up with the belief that food is 'dangerous' or the enemy; food can still be fun, delicious and satisfying, no matter how many allergies your child has.

Coping with an allergic child
Education
Education is the key, and your child will need to understand his condition, and know how important it is to avoid problem foods. You don't need to scare him, but you do need to present the risks in a way that will make him understand the potential severity. Try not to make him feel 'different'.

Simply point out that he has special requirements, and show him how to be diligent. This involves not swapping food at school, avoiding things like buffets, takeaway or restaurant food, and even school meals.

Younger children

Younger children will obviously not be able to make informed choices or decisions, so you will need to advise other parents, teachers, carers and friends about the situation, and pre-plan. If your child is unable to eat the foods his friends are eating, find out in advance what's being served and see if you can produce something similar. Even very young children can be taught not to take food from others, or from other people's plates. Your child doesn't need to feel different; turn it around and make out that your child is 'special' and has her own 'special food'.

Family meals

Most toddlers and young children want to be involved in family meals, and to eat what everyone else is eating. It is not hard to adapt an allergen-free diet for the whole family. For dairy sufferers, use olive oil or vegan margarines in cooking instead of butter; breads containing a variety of other grains are now readily available and can be enjoyed by the whole family; offer cheese, seeds and nuts on the side; substitute non-wheat pastas for your allergic child; serve baked or fresh fruits for desserts instead of problematic puddings. If the whole family is sitting down to scrambled eggs, scramble up a little tofu with herbs. It is not as hard as you think, and you'll find the whole family may well eat better as a result.

School

Send a supply of 'safe' snacks with your child to school, and teach her not to swap. Talk to your child's school about what foods are suitable and ensure that there is plenty of 'safe' food on the menu. If you are concerned, send a packed lunch. Above all, and once again, teach your child what she can and can't eat and explain what can

must know
Recognizing an allergic reaction
Teach your child and his teachers to recognize the signs of an allergic reaction. It is one thing to educate others on treatment, but if they don't know what to look for, it may well be too late. Since you can't be with your child at all times, it is important for him and the adults around him to be aware of the allergy and be alert for signs of it.

happen if she is tempted to eat the wrong foods. Consider requesting a 'peanut ban' if your child is severely allergic.

Make your child's school aware of any allergies. Write a letter and highlight the specific foods in bold, or in a different colour ink. Send copies to your child's teacher, school nurse, head teacher and any-one else who deals with him on a regular basis. Ask your child's teacher what projects (in art, or the science lab, for example) might contain foods that could cause a reaction. Find an alternative well in advance.

Everyone who may come into contact with the child should be informed of his/her food allergies. Depending on the extent of the child's food allergies, he may have to sit at a separate table in the cafeteria during lunchtime. If the child's allergies are very severe, he may have to eat in a separate room away from the other pupils, or near the teacher's desk.

Make sure your child and/or the school has access to emergency treatment (an EpiPen, for example, see page 102), and that everyone involved learns how to recognize symptoms and knows how to administer treatment. Older children can be taught to administer epinephrine themselves. Make sure your child has an allergy alert bracelet, or something on his person explaining his allergies. If he or she experiences an attack while away from people who are aware of the situation, this crucial information may save his life.

want to know more?

For information on food additives and their effect on children's behaviour, as well as information on food labelling, visit the Food Standards Agency, at www.food.gov.uk/ safereating/allergyintol.

Allergy UK offers a wealth of tips for keeping your allergic child safe and healthy. Visit: www.allergyuk.org.

Kidsaware is a unique site that sells 'allergy awareness' products for children, such as 'nut allergy' lunchboxes and personalised allergy labels. Visit www.kidsaware.co.uk.

If your child suffers from severe reactions, you'll benefit from the wealth of information at the Anaphylaxis Campaign; site has food alerts, plenty of tips, product information and guidance for schools. Visit www.anaphylaxis.org.uk, or ring 01252 542029.

Case study

Mandy

Mandy had been a difficult baby, with colic, frequent night-time wakings, and consistent crying. When she reached toddlerhood, she became a terror – running all the time, jumping, talking incessantly, and throwing wild tantrums when she didn't get what she wanted. She had been formula-fed from birth, and her behaviour didn't seem to become obviously worse when she started solid food, so her parents were surprised to learn that there might be a link to food allergies. Mandy did, however, suffer from frequent skin rashes, abdominal pain, headaches, and she had the classic 'circles' around her eyes that many 'allergic' or 'intolerant' children have. When she started school, she had difficulty concentrating, said she couldn't 'hear' the teacher, and became extremely disruptive, causing chaos in an otherwise quiet class. In desperation, Mandy's parents agreed to try Ritalin, which left her much calmer, but did nothing to abate any of the other symptoms. A friend recommended a nutritionist, who took one look at Mandy and suggested that food allergies might be at the root of the problem. She discovered that Mandy's diet centred almost entirely around milk and wheat – cereal, cheese sandwiches, pasta with cheese, pizza – as well as a number of sweetened products, such as biscuits, cakes, fizzy drinks, sweets, chocolate and a great deal of concentrated fruit juice. Mandy was put on a 'caveman' diet, with no grains apart from rice, no dairy produce, no citrus fruit, and no additives, preservatives or sugar. The first night on this programme Mandy was up all night screaming in pain, and crying – she vomited, had pains in her stomach and couldn't sleep. In alarm her parents called the nutritionist, who told them that Mandy was suffering withdrawal symptoms. For the next few days she was moody and irritable, lacking energy, and sleeping poorly, but on the sixth day, she was a new child. Allergy tests later showed that she was intolerant to both dairy produce and wheat (the former of which had started her problems in infancy); she was also sensitive to a variety of different food additives, and naturally occurring salicylates. What's more, Mandy had a high sensitivity to sugar. Mandy's diet was adapted to take into consideration her nutritional needs and the foods that had to be avoided. Now ten years old, she has stopped taking Ritalin completely, and is, her parents say, a completely different child – calmer, happier and relaxed.

6 Allergic illness

The link between a number of health conditions and allergic reactions has become clear over the past decades, and more and more 'diseases' are considered to be 'allergic illnesses' – that is, they are caused or exacerbated by allergies and tend to occur in allergic or atopic people. Asthma, hay fever and eczema are three atopic diseases that are characterized by an excess production of antibody IgE, which causes the symptoms. But other conditions, such as coeliac disease, irritable bowel syndrome, thrush, migraine and even rheumatism may also have an allergic root.

Coeliac disease

Coeliac disease is a condition caused by an inability to digest gluten, which often manifests itself in bowel problems and weight loss or failure to gain weight. Gluten, a protein in wheat, barley, oats and rye, reacts with the small intestine, and causes damage by activating the immune system to attack the delicate lining of the bowel.

must know
Coelic disease
Some people are genetically predisposed to coeliac disease. The result is that sub-sections of the proteins found in wheat, gluten and gliadin, become toxic to the lining of the gut. A blood test can test for antibodies against gluten and gliadin. If the blood test is abnormal, your doctor will arrange for you to see a gastro-enterologist, who is likely to organize taking specimens from the small intestine. If gluten has been eaten the intestine will typically have a worn-down appearance, which returns to normal after a period of excluding it from the diet. It is therefore important to stay on a normal diet until after the biopsy so that you will get an accurate result.

In the bowel there are long finger-like protrusions, which increase the bowel's surface area and allow the maximum number of nutrients, vitamins and minerals to be absorbed. In coeliac disease, these protrusions are destroyed, meaning that nutrients pass down along the intestines without being absorbed. As a result, anaemia, osteoporosis, poor growth and even some cancers may result, if the condition is untreated.

If the condition is left untreated, the disease can cause serious effects. For example, as nutrients are absorbed in insufficient quantities from the bowel, there may be weight loss or, in children, a failure to thrive or grow. Sufferers may have a swollen or bloated abdomen. Secondary symptoms, such as anaemia, may cause shortness of breath or fatigue. The first symptom is often irritability and poor appetite, combined with weight loss. Some children start it with vomiting and diarrhoea, so it can be wrongly diagnosed as gastoenteritis. A child's stomach may become swollen, and the muscles of his arms and legs become wasted and thin. Secondary symptoms, such as anaemia, may cause shortness of breath or fatigue.

The condition is often diagnosed in childhood after weaning when cereals are introduced into the diet, although it can be diagnosed at any age. The symptoms can be subtle, so that you may feel unwell for no reason for some time before the diagnosis is made.

Treatment

The only really successful treatment for coeliac disease is to exclude gluten from your diet for the remainder of your life. It is not as difficult as it may seem, as food labelling has improved a great deal, and there are many gluten-free alternatives now available.

Gluten, a substance found in wheat, oats, barley and rye, reacts with the small bowel, causing damage by activating the immune system to attack the delicate lining of the bowel, which is responsible for absorbing nutrients and vitamins.

Living with coeliac disease

Although coeliac disease is not preventable, sticking to a gluten-free diet can reverse damage to the small intestine. Gluten occurs in bread, biscuits, cakes and pastries, pasta, breakfast cereals and is also used in some manufactured soups and sauces. Gluten is also 'hidden' in some foods such as crisps and similar snacks, as well as chips in restaurants. Some vegetable oils may contain wheatgerm oil, and malt vinegar, soya sauce, mustard and mayonnaise also contain gluten. Oats do contain a small amount of gluten, but many sufferers can tolerate them; however, because they are often milled and stored in the same mills as wheat, they may be contaminated with gluten.

There are plenty of foods that do not contain gluten, including all fruit, vegetables, rice, corn, nuts, potatoes, red meat, poultry, fish, eggs, pulses and dairy produce. And the growing number of gluten-free substitute products is also growing, including gluten-free breads, pastas, biscuits, cereals and other baked goods. See page 41 for details of foods containing gluten, and ideas for replacing crucial nutrients that may be lost by excluding wheat from your diet.

did you know?

Until recently, it was believed that coeliac disease only occurs in about one in 1,500 people. It is now thought to be more common; more accurate testing methods show that about one in 300 people in the UK, Europe and USA suffer from this condition. If you have a parent, sibling or child with coeliac disease, you have a 10 per cent chance of also developing it. If you have an identical twin with coeliac disease, your chances are increased to more than 70 per cent.

Lactose intolerance

Like coeliac disease, lactose intolerance is not an allergy as such, but an inability of the body to break down lactose, the sugar in milk. The substance produced by the body for this purpose is called lactase, and sufferers have insufficient quantities to allow them to digest lactose.

Symptoms can be painful, and include cramps, bloating, gas, diarrhoea and sometimes nausea, which may begin half an hour to two hours after eating or drinking foods containing lactose. The severity of symptoms varies depending on the amount of lactose each individual can tolerate. Some of the symptoms may be similar to those of a milk allergy but milk allergies can cause the body to react more quickly, more often within a few minutes. It is worth comparing the symptoms of a true milk allergy (see page 27) with those of lactose intolerance so that you are clear.

Lactose intolerance has a high genetic basis, and is a common feature of many races, including Asian, African, some Mediterranean countries, and native populations of Canada, US, Australia and New Zealand. It may also be temporary, following an illness effecting the gut, a long course of antibiotics, or injury to the intestines.

Unless it is a temporary condition, which normally resolves itself within a week, lactose intolerance is not curable. There are two ways to cope with lactose intolerance. The first is to avoid dairy produce completely, unless it is lactose-free. Some sufferers can tolerate small amounts of lactose, so lactose-reduced milks, cheeses and other produce may also be acceptable. It is important, too, to look for hidden sources of milk (see page 30).

The second coping method is to replace the lactase that your digestive system is not producing. This way you may be able to enjoy dairy products without any symptoms. There is a handful of pharmaceutical companies that produce lactase enzyme tablets to take with food; there are also lactase enzyme drops to treat milk (see page 27).

Diagnosing lactose intolerance

There are three main ways to test for lactose intolerance: the lactose tolerance test, the hydrogen breath test, and the stool acidity test.

• *The lactose tolerance test* begins with fasting (not eating) before the test and then drinking a liquid that contains lactose. Several blood samples are taken over a two-hour period to measure your blood glucose (blood sugar) level, which indicates how well the body is able to digest lactose.
• *The hydrogen breath test* measures the amount of hydrogen in the breath. Normally, very little hydrogen is detectable in the breath. However, undigested lactose in the colon is fermented by bacteria, and various gases, including hydrogen, are produced. The hydrogen is absorbed from the intestines, carried through the bloodstream to the lungs, and exhaled. In the test, you drink a lactose-loaded beverage, and your breath is analyzed at regular intervals.
• *A stool acidity test*, which measures the amount of acid in the stool, may be given to babies and young children (who are rarely given the first two tests because of concerns about overloading them with lactose). Undigested lactose fermented by bacteria in the colon creates lactic acid and other acids that can be detected in a stool sample. In addition, glucose may be present in the sample as a result of unabsorbed lactose in the colon.

Eczema

The most common type of eczema is known as 'atopic eczema', and it often appears as patches of reddish, scaling skin. As eczema worsens, the skin becomes itchier, red, thickened, grooved, and may blister, weep and crack. It is typically found on the face, behind the ears, on the front of the elbows, the back of the knees, the hands, neck, and trunk.

did you know?

Atopic eczema affects about ten to 20 per cent of schoolchildren and three to five per cent of adults in the UK. Over the last 30 years, eczema has more than quadrupled. It seems likely though that increasing exposure to allergens (protein substances to which people can become allergic) such as house dust mites and other environmental factors have been the main causes of this increase. The good news is that half of all children outgrow eczema by the age of six, two thirds outgrow it by 14, and only one-third of all cases persist into adulthood.

Food allergy probably accounts for most eczema suffering; the rest is the result of external allergy-irritants, infection, and injury to the skin through vigorous itching. House dust mite allergy is an important external cause of eczema. Infection with the bacteria staphylococci is a common cause of sudden worsening of eczema.

Atopic eczema is linked with the family of allergies that includes hay fever and asthma, and is most commonly linked with food allergies. In fact, cow's milk allergy is often the cause of severe and widespread eczema. Up to a third of infantile eczema is food allergy related and food additives and colourings may also aggravate eczema in older children. In addition adverse reactions to citrus fruit, tomatoes, pineapples and Marmite, are common in people with eczema. In a nutshell, however, any food or substance can cause eczema if there is an allergy and you are susceptible.

Children commonly outgrow eczema, particularly if the triggers (food allergies, for example) are dealt with; although they can relapse in adulthood. If the condition begins in adulthood, it is not usually outgrown, although it can certainly be controlled.

There are several types of eczema, atopic eczema being the most common. Other types include contact eczema (or dermatitis) which appears when the skin comes into contact with an allergen, or an irritant, such as an acid, cleaning product or other chemical. This does not tend to have an allergic basis, although allergic people tend to be more sensitive. Allergic contact eczema (or dermatitis) is a red, itchy, weepy reaction that occurs when the skin comes into contact with something that the immune system recognizes as foreign, such as chemicals in creams and lotions or poison ivy. Seborrhoeic eczema is a form of skin inflammation that appears as yellowish, oily, scaly patches of skin on the scalp, face, and occasionally other parts of the body. Cradle cap in newborn babies is a type of seborrhoeic eczema. The cause of this is largely unknown but, once again, it does seem more common in atopic children and adults.

Treating eczema

Getting to the root cause of eczema is the most important part of the treatment, and involves identifying the allergens that may be triggering it. Foods are an important first place to start, and you can begin by keeping a food diary (see page 72), and then going on to an elimination diet (see page 82). Skin prick or blood tests will confirm the problem foods (see page 77). Avoiding the problem foods is the best way to keep eczema under control, and total abstinence is important. Although flare-ups may not be life threatening, you have more chance of outgrowing or 'curing' the condition if you avoid allergenic foods completely for as long as possible. Even then, during periods of ill health, or when you are stressed, run down or have taken a course of antibiotics, the condition can flare up again.

must know
Eczema
While researchers are uncertain of the exact processes involved, eczema is largely considered an allergic disease. 80 per cent of all eczema patients have higher than normal levels of the antibody immunoglobulin E (IgE). Such skin has a tendency to be 'overgrown' with bacteria, mainly staphylococcus aureus. For this reason, many people respond to antibacterial emollients, which not only prevent secondary infection, but keep the skin clear. This may also explain why treatment with probiotics (see page 185) can help both to prevent and address cases.

Similarly, moulds, dust mites, and other allergens possibly causing the problem can be tested for, and removed, as much as possible, from your environment. Probiotics, which are 'healthy' bacteria, can be taken to recolonize the gut and regain a balance between healthy and unhealthy bacteria. In some studies, this has proved to be successful in keeping eczema under control – largely, perhaps, because the gut is implicated in so many cases.

Your doctor can also recommend treatments that will keep eczema under control, although these will do little to address the root cause:

• *Emollients* are moisturizing creams, ointments and bath additives and are the mainstay of eczema treatment. They are used to hydrate and protect the skin. *Cortisone or steroid creams* produce quick relief of symptoms and can be used for short periods, during flare-ups. Long-term use may lead to thinning of the skin.

• *Wet wraps* are applied at night to retain moisture in the skin, aid absorption of creams and to protect against scratching. First of all, emollients and steroid creams are applied to the affected areas. Elasticated cotton-based tubular dressings are soaked in warm water and then cut to size so that they cover the affected areas. These can be applied overnight to the limbs, trunk, neck and even face (holes are cut in the dressing to allow for eyes, ears, nose and mouth). This treatment is highly successful for severe weepy eczema.

• *Antibiotics*: Eczema sufferers are more prone to skin infections such as bacterial, fungal and viral infections, including the common wart). Antibiotic creams and occasionally oral antibiotics are prescribed to treat infected eczema, which may suddenly crust and ooze.

• *Antihistamines*: tablets or syrups reduce itching, especially at night. Antihistamine creams may sensitize the skin and should be avoided.

must know
Evening primrose oil
This has been used successfully in the treatment of eczema, reducing itching and encouraging healing. A study carried out by the Department of Dermatology at Bristol's Royal Infirmary showed a significant improvement in those with atopic eczema. These improvements were recorded after just three weeks of taking 400mg of evening primrose oil a day (200mg for children). The evening primrose oil was shown to lessen itching by 36 per cent, scaling by 33 per cent and redness by 29 per cent.

Asthma

Asthma is the third in the trilogy of atopic allergic illnesses, which also includes asthma, eczema and hay fever. Asthma, a chronic medical condition, effects more than five per cent of the population, although many studies show this to be a very conservative estimate (see box below).

Asthma results when triggers (or irritants) cause swelling of the tissues to the air passages of the lungs, making it difficult to breathe. Typical symptoms of asthma include wheezing, coughing, and shortness of breath.

Asthma can be triggered by numerous factors, including allergens from dust, moulds, pollen, animals and food; air pollutants, such as cigarette smoke, auto exhaust, smog, or aerosol cleaners; colds and particularly respiratory infections; weather changes; exercise; or certain medications.

The food allergy link

Many studies of food allergy involve people with food-induced asthma. The asthma is easily recognized if symptoms begin within a few hours of eating food and the asthma is associated with other symptoms of food allergy. Atopic people with food allergies are also more likely to have eczema and asthma together. For example, one study found that in a group of 320 kids with eczema, more than half also had asthma, and food allergies caused asthmatic symptoms in almost 60 per cent of them. Unfortunately, asthma is often treated only as an airborne allergy problem or as a problem unrelated to allergic processes and the possible role of food allergy is neglected. Part of the problem may also be the fact that the reaction is

did you know?
A recent study shows that the number of children suffering from asthma has risen dramatically in the last decade. A survey of 3,000 children aged six and seven found that 23 per cent of them had suffered from asthma at some point in their lives, up from 13 per cent when a previous study was carried out. The UK has among the highest incidence of asthma, which has increased 30 times over the last 30 years.

delayed in some people (delayed pattern food allergy), which means that the foods triggering the asthma are not usually picked up with skin prick or blood tests. Many cases of chronic asthma are blamed on this type of food allergy. Sometimes certain foods are identified in chronic asthmatics, but many others may not be, simply because symptoms do not manifest themselves until much later (even days after ingesting the food).

In reality, allergy can cause both immediate and delayed patterns of asthma. Immediate food reactions can cause sudden, dramatic and life-threatening asthma and it is one of the consequences of anaphylactic reactions to food (see pages 101-102).

Both IgE and non-IgE mechanisms can cause asthma. Studies show that asthma sufferers with no positive skin tests can still react to foods. Several landmark pieces of research show that milk, wheat, egg, yeast, preservatives, colourings, coffee, salicylates and cheese are the main foods implicated, and found that other manifestations of food allergy are typical in 65 per cent of the asthmatics.

Treating asthma

The best way to avoid food-induced asthma is to eliminate or avoid the offending food or food ingredient from the diet or from the environment. Get used to reading food labels and become familiar with your own food triggers. Once again, a food diary, a simple elimination diet, and some conventional testing should root out the offending foods. However, in the case of delayed pattern food allergies, you will need to reintroduce foods one and at a time, and wait at least five days before

> **must know**
> **Asthma triggers**
> Sulphites and sulphiting agents in foods (found in dried fruits, prepared potatoes, wine, bottled lemon or lime juice, and prawns, for example), and diagnosed food allergens (such as milk, eggs, peanuts, tree nuts, soya, wheat, fish, and shellfish) have been found to trigger asthma. Many food ingredients such as food dyes and colours, food preservatives like BHA and BHT, monosodium glutamate (MSG), aspartame, and nitrites, have not been conclusively linked to asthma, but they have been shown to cause problems in susceptible people.

introducing another – noting any asthmatic symptoms as they appear.

There are some useful tips on page 101 for making your environment less allergenic. These measures are invaluable for asthmatics, as all seem to have at least some allergic response to things like pollen, moulds, animal fur or dust mites.

Conventional treatment is with two types of drug: relieving drugs and preventing drugs.

The relieving drugs such as salbutamol (Ventolin) and terbutaline (Bricanyl) act within minutes to open the airways and bring relief from symptoms, but wear off within a few hours and fail to deal with the underlying inflammation of the airways.

Preventing drugs such as beclo-methasone (Becotide), budesonide (Pulmicort), or sodium chromoglycate (Intal) tackle the root of the problem – the inflammation in the airways. They act slowly over several hours and their full effect may not be apparent for several days. These drugs are used regularly, whether you are well or ill, in order to keep the inflammation at bay and prevent long-term or permanent damage to the airways.

If your asthma symptoms become severe, your doctor or asthma nurse may give you a short course (three to 14 days) of steroid tablets. Steroid tablets work quickly and powerfully to help to calm your inflamed airways. Short courses of steroid tablets are also used to treat acute asthma attacks and are used for any essential emergency treatment of asthma attacks.

must know
Causes of asthma
The causes are still largely unknown. Apart from the link to food allergies, we do know that younger siblings in a family are less likely than older siblings to get asthma – possibly because they build up a healthy immunity by being in contact with more infections (and dirt!) through family members. So it follows that aspects of modern lifestyles – such as changes in housing and diet and a more hygienic environment – may have contributed to the rise in asthma over the last few decades. Research has shown that smoking during pregnancy significantly increases the risk of a child developing asthma, and children whose parents smoke are more likely to develop asthma. Adult-onset asthma may develop after a viral infection.

Irritable bowel syndrome

Irritable bowel syndrome (IBS) affects approximately ten to 15 per cent or more of the general population; in fact, it is the most common disease diagnosed by gastroenterologists (doctors who specialize in treating the stomach and intestines). Sometimes irritable bowel syndrome is referred to as spastic colon, mucous colitis, spastic colitis, nervous stomach or irritable colon.

Although not strictly an allergic illness, food allergies and sensitivities to certain foods are implicated in many, many cases. In people with IBS, symptoms result from what appears to be a disturbance in the interaction between the gut or intestines, the brain, and the autonomic nervous system that alters regulation of bowel motility (motor function) or sensory function. Irritable bowel syndrome is characterized by a group of symptoms in which abdominal pain or discomfort is associated with a change in bowel pattern, such as loose or more frequent bowel movements, diarrhoea, and/or constipation.

Certain foods are known to stimulate gut reactions in general, and in those with IBS eating too much of these might cause or make symptoms worse. For example, meals that are too large or high in fat, fried foods, coffee, caffeine, or alcohol may provoke symptoms of abdominal cramps and diarrhoea. Eating too much of some types of sugar that are poorly absorbed by the bowel can also cause cramping or diarrhoea. Some foods are gas producing (for example, beans, cabbage, pulses, cauliflower, broccoli, lentils, Brussels sprouts, raisins, onions, and bagels) and eating too much may cause increased gas, particularly as IBS can be associated with retention of gas and bloating.

What about food allergies?

A 2005 study found that 65 per cent of IBS sufferers believed that food allergies were at the root of their condition, and researchers found that IBS patients have raised levels of antibodies to foods such as wheat, beef, pork, lamb and soya bean, among others. What's more, two thirds of IBS sufferers have been found to have hidden food intolerances. The worst culprits are wheat, dairy, coffee, tea, citrus fruits, and lactose

Common trigger foods

These are not necessarily foods to which you are allergic, but which are known to cause symptoms in a large number of IBS sufferers:

alcohol	fizzy drinks
artificial sweeteners	fried foods
chocolate	oils
coconut milk	poultry skin and dark
coffee (even decaffeinated)	meat
dairy	red meat
egg yolks	

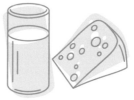

Foods that may cause gas

bananas	garlic
beans	leeks
broccoli	nuts
sprouts	onions
cabbage	raisins
cauliflower	

Foods that may cause sensitivities

sorbitol (a sugar substitute)

fructose (found in fruit juice and dried fruit)

lactose (found in milk)

wheat bran

IBS treatment
Your doctor may
prescribe laxatives for a
limited period, if
constipation is a
regular problem;
however, these do
nothing to address
bloating and gas.
Antispasmodic
medicines relieve the
stomach cramps
brought on by IBS by
relaxing the smooth
muscle of the gut. But
they also may cause
constipation, so they
aren't usually
prescribed for people
who suffer IBS with
constipation. Some
doctors offer
antidepressants, not
because depression is
necessarily a feature,
but because these
drugs interfere with the
brain's perception of
gut pain.

(the sugar in cow's milk). In 20 per cent of sufferers, potatoes are a problem too. An elimination diet that removes these foods has been shown to help.

In fact, most sufferers know of one or two foods that can bring on symptoms. Whether these are full-blown allergies or intolerance, or merely sensitivities, is often unknown, as symptoms can often manifest themselves even days after eating problematic foods.

Treating IBS

Using the methods to detect a food allergy or intolerance, which we discussed earlier in this book (see page 72) would be a good first port of call. If you can rule out foods that set off your symptoms, avoidance is the obvious choice of treatment and can be very effective. Some sufferers are able to return to eating problematic foods after several months of avoiding them. Remember, however, that in many cases, intolerance or sensitivities may be at the root of your IBS rather than true allergies, so ensure that you wait at least four or five days to note any symptoms, as they may take that long to manifest themselves.

If you don't get anywhere, you may require allergy testing, although this is not particularly effective for intolerance or sensitivities. The only really reliable tool for diagnosis is a properly managed elimination diet. You may also want to consider whether lactose may be the problem (see page 156).

Eating several smaller meals during the day, rather than three large ones, may also help to reduce symptoms. Some people with IBS find that large meals may result in cramping and diarrhoea. Additionally, many people find it helpful to keep their meals low in fat, and high in carbohydrates such as whole-grain breads, pasta, rice, fruits, vegetables, and cereals.

In some cases, fibre is another important element of treatment, as it may help to prevent spasms by keeping the colon distended. It also absorbs water, which helps to prevent constipation. A high-fibre diet must also be accompanied by plenty of fresh water – at least eight big glasses a day. Good sources of fibre include flaxseeds, bran, whole grains, pulses, rice, fruit and vegetables (particularly with their skins on), and seeds. Some sufferers experience problems with fibre, so talk to your specialist or nutritionist to work out what is best for you.

Lactobacillus acidophilus, a probiotic, or 'friendly bacteria' may be helpful in aiding digestion. Acidophilus helps to maintain the 'good' bacteria in the gut. It is readily found in yoghurt that contains live cultures. Yoghurt contains calcium, and is by and large better tolerated than other milk products due to the active cultures. Natural probiotics include bananas, onions, garlic, artichokes, barley, rye, tomatoes, honey, and asparagus - but if you have IBS you will probably find it difficult to eat enough to make a big difference. Probiotic drinks, such as Actimel and Yakult, taken two or three times a day, can improve symptoms.

did you know?
Studies at Addenbrooke's Hospital in Cambridge found that of 182 IBS patients, dietary changes were able to completely relieve symptoms in 122 cases. So don't give up!

Other conditions

Many other health conditions may be linked to allergies to some extent, including rheumatoid arthritis, psoriasis and urticaria. It is beyond the scope of this book to examine them all, but let's look at the links.

Arthritis

Rheumatoid arthritis is a chronic disease in which the joints holding two or more bones together become inflamed and cause pain, stiffness, and swelling. Eventually, these affected joints become deformed. Rheumatoid arthritis most commonly affects the joints in the hands and feet, as well as the shoulders, jaw, hips, and knees. Rheumatoid arthritis is a type of autoimmune disease where our body's immune cells attack and kill what they see as foreign invaders, usually bacteria, viruses, and fungi. However, with autoimmune diseases, something needs to trigger the immune system to perceive the body's own tissues as foreign invaders.

Some researchers believe certain people are more likely to develop an autoimmune disease as a result of their genetic make-up, and all it takes is some type of infection to trigger the immune system to spiral out of control. Autoimmune disorders have also been linked to food allergies. Some people with rheumatoid arthritis find they have flare-ups after eating certain foods. While there is some evidence that food allergies play a role in the overall severity of symptoms, it is unclear whether food allergies are the cause or the result of an overactive intestinal immune system.

Migraine

A migraine is a moderate to severe headache usually on one side of the head. However, migraine headaches can occur on different sides of the same migraine sufferer at different times. Migraine causes sharp pain that usually throbs and patients with migraine usually lose their appetite, feel nauseous and may vomit. The symptoms can be so intense that many sufferers can do little but lie down in a darkened room.

Although migraine has not usually been considered an allergic condition, there is no doubt that allergies play a part to some extent. For example, almost all sufferers can list a food or two that triggers their migraine; common culprits include sulphites, red wine, nuts, aspartame, chocolate, MSG, caffeine, nitrates, spinach, dairy produce and wheat. Symptoms do not occur every time these foods are eaten, but they are often a cause of them when they do occur. This obviously rules out a true food allergy; however, but it does suggest sensitivity or intolerance that, in combination with other factors, such as stress, lack of sleep or hormonal activity, for example, can cause problems.

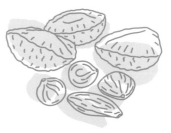

Interestingly, too, studies show that allergies, asthma and migraine are linked. If you inherit one of these disorders, you have a greater likelihood of inheriting one or more of the others. In a recent study, 40 to 70 per cent of migraine sufferers reported having allergies. Other studies have reported that people with migraine are two to three and a half times more likely to have asthma, particularly if they have a parent with migraine and asthma. Therefore, the link between allergies (including those to food) and migraine is currently the subject of much research.

watch out!
Dehydration is often a precursor to migraine, as is stress. Keeping well hydrated as well as taking time to relax, is as important as any dietary changes.

Treating migraine

Your doctor will undoubtedly offer anti-nausea medication, painkillers, or anti-migraine drugs that dampen the migraine process itself by altering the activity of chemical 'messengers' in the brain and perhaps altering blood flow as well.

Although true food allergy may not be at the root, it is a good idea to keep a food diary and note which foods trigger or cause your symptoms. Note, too, any other symptoms, including digestive disturbances, sleep problems, mood, skin rashes and your breathing. It would also help to switch to a healthy low-allergen diet (see page 141) for a period of time, to see if your symptoms abate. If you find that this makes a difference, it is worth consulting a nutritionist or allergy specialist who can help you to work out which foods really are problematic, and which can be safely reintroduced. It may well be that sensitivities to the chemicals in foods (particularly those that are processed) may be the culprits, which simply means keeping this type of food to a minimum.

Although migraines are not life threatening, they can be disruptive and extremely debilitating. You can likely take risks with food sensitivities, knowing you will pay for that glass of red wine or bacon sandwich later, but being aware of your problem foods is the best preventative medicine of all.

Psoriasis

Psoriasis is a chronic skin disorder that effects about two per cent of the population. It is characterized by red, elevated plaques that are often overlaid with thick, silvery white scales. The most commonly affected affected areas are the elbows, knees, scalp, lower back,

watch out!

Exercising after eating certain foods such as wheat, celery and shellfish might provoke delayed urticaria.

and genitalia. Some people have psoriasis on their hands and feet. There is a definite genetic predisposition for psoriasis. When one parent is affected, there is roughly a ten per cent risk of a child acquiring psoriasis. The risk rises to almost 50 per cent when both parents have psoriasis. One study analyzing psoriasis in twins found there was a 65 per cent chance of identical twin siblings having psoriasis when the other twin was affected. The exact mode of inheritance is complex and variable. The National Psoriasis Foundation reported that researchers have discovered evidence that psoriasis is an autoimmune disorder. What is more, many sufferers appear to be sensitive (although possibly not allergic) to a number of foods, including gluten, food additives, and the 'nightshade' vegetables: potatoes, tomatoes, bell peppers and aubergine. It is worth having it checked out; if maybe not the cause, food allergies or intolerance can certainly promote flare-ups in some people. Some studies indicate that oily fish can improve the condition; however, the quantity required to make substantial improvements is very high. Under the supervision of your doctor, you may wish to try taking fish oil capsules.

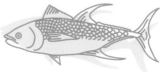

Urticaria

Urticaria, or hives, is a common symptom of food allergies, and usually appears fairly instantly upon eating problematic foods. It is characterized by itchy, elevated, red blotches of varying size that appear suddenly and disappear mysteriously after hours to days.

In cases of intolerance or sensitivities, urticaria can appear later on (as long as 48 hours after eating suspect foods). Acute (sudden) urticaria is almost always caused by an allergy to food (or another substance) and can last between several hours and six weeks. Chronic urticaria is

Candida

Overgrowth of candida yeast in the digestive tract or mucous membranes, called candidiasis, was popularized by William Crook, MD, in his 1983 book, *The Yeast Connection*. While some doctors dismiss candidiasis as a 'fad' diagnosis, an increasing number of doctors and naturopaths are recognizing that a candida infection can be a serious health concern. While not a symptom of food allergy in most people, candida may be a trigger of symptoms and a cause of food allergies. It is also considered in some quarters to be an allergy to yeast.

Candida albicans occurs naturally in the gut, in the skin and in the vagina. Under normal circumstances, it is kept under control by other 'friendly' bacteria in the body, but occasionally it overgrows, which is when problems start. Common causes of overgrowth include:
- taking antibiotics
- natural hormonal changes (for example, during pregnancy, around your period, or during menopause)
- taking hormones such as the pill or HRT
- becoming run down (by overwork, for example)
- suffering from continual stress
- a compromised immune system (you may feel that you are always 'coming down with something')
- undiagnosed or poorly controlled diabetes
- sex with someone who has thrush
- long-term steroid use

When antibiotics are given for infection, they do not discriminate between the 'good' bacteria and the 'bad' bacteria in the body. They wipe out everything, which means that there is not enough of the 'good' bacteria to keep fungi (and other 'invaders') such as thrush at bay. What's the result? Candida is no longer controlled and it begins to overgrow.

The theory is that candida can inflame the colon, contribute to leaky gut syndrome, effect the body's immunity, which causes hostile reactions to foods, and generally leads to poor health, which could be a contributing factor to food allergies. There is no doubt that candida can overgrow, but the extent to which it is affected by or effects food allergies is still unclear.

diagnosed if the rash persists for six weeks or longer. The latter is less likely to be due to a true food allergy, but may involve food additives such as salicylates, sodium benzoate, colourings and nitrates.

Atopic children with eczema and rhinitis are prone to urticaria from food. Urticaria is associated with high IgE and occurs usually as an acute food reactions. It also occurs as a feature of anaphylactic reactions. Infants may develop facial weals on contact with food. Adults often have a single bout of hives when they encounter an unusual or seasonal food or take a drug.

want to know more?

Greens Foods has a good range of supplements for allergic illnesses, including probiotics and prebiotics. Contact them on 0800 0937 615 or 020 7222 5902, or visit www.greensfoods.co.uk.

Support organizations that may be of use include: the National Eczema Society (www.eczema.org; 020 7281 3553); the Candida Society (www.candida-society.org; 01689 813039); the IBS Network (www.ibsnetwork.org.uk; 0114 2723253); Asthma UK (www.asthma.org.uk; 020 72262260) and the British Lung Foundation (www.lunguk.org; 020 7831 5831).

For information on all aspects of food allergies and allergic illnesses that may be food-linked, contact Allergy UK on their helpline: 01322 619898, or visit www.allergyuk.org.

An organization called Allergy-induced Autism offers an excellent overview of leaky gut syndrome, with plenty of advice. Visit www.autismmedical.com.

7 Preventing allergies

Suffering from food allergies is not a life sentence, and it does not mean giving up all the pleasures of good food. Avoiding foods that cause a reaction can make a huge difference to your life, and the more scrupulous you are about keeping them out of your diet, the more likely you are to outgrow them. More importantly, perhaps, there is no reason to assume that your children will suffer the same or greater allergies, no matter the odds stacked against them. A great deal of research has been undertaken into the science of allergy prevention. Let's look at what can make a difference.

The genetic link

Food allergies run in families, and evidence appears to support the idea that food intolerances do as well. For example, a 2000 study found that peanut allergies are inherited in 87 per cent of cases; if both parents suffer from allergies, children have a 40 per cent chance of being allergic – and if both parents suffer from the same allergies, the risk increases to more than 70 per cent. More than half of all children with food allergies have at least one parent with food allergies or allergic disease.

must know
Pregnancy and allergies
Allergies sometimes appear for the first time in pregnancy, due to hormonal changes and stress on the body's systems; however, an elimination diet should never be undertaken without the supervision of an allergy specialist. Pregnancy requires optimum nutrition to ensure the health of mother and baby. Nevertheless, you should always be scrupulous in avoiding any foods to which you have a known food allergy – particularly if your reactions involve anaphylaxis.

So the odds seem stacked against some children from day one. Can anything be done to prevent allergies?

Pregnancy

There is conflicting research into this one, but several studies show some interesting results. One study found that removing peanuts from your diet during pregnancy can help to prevent peanut allergy in your child. Indeed, some researchers see a benefit to eliminating the type of allergen that has a high potential for causing serious allergies; for example, if there is a strong fish or shellfish allergy in the family, it is probably sensible to avoid these foods during pregnancy. However, there were less conclusive results with eggs and dairy produce, and many experts believe that removing these from your your diet during pregnancy may compromise nutrition and affect the health of you and your baby. The wealth of research does, however, point to the fact that the risk of developing allergies in infancy does not decrease when you avoid allergenic foods.

Too little is known about allergies to make it clean cut and your diet will not suffer if you drop one or two highly allergenic foods.

To confuse the issue further, a recent study found that some babies can be sensitized to foods before they are born, because some food molecules from the food eaten by their mothers can reach the womb. The foods most likely to cause problems are often those craved by women while they were pregnant, or foods that were eaten in large quantities. This may suggest an intolerance or sensitivity in the pregnant mother (cravings can be a sign of intolerance, see page 85), which may then make her baby more likely to be allergic. The sensible approach is to avoid overeating any one food, and to work out if the foods you are craving are causing any other symptoms – lethargy, headaches, irritability, for example. An elimination diet is not appropriate for pregnant women, so simply cut down on the foods that may be problematic, or see a specialist if you suspect an allergy. Some women crave foods that will supply them with nutrients missing in their diet; however, a good, balanaced diet with no over-emphasis on any one food will ensure that nutritional needs are met. Finally, current evidence is inconclusive regarding the effect of a pregnant mother's diet on her baby. The only strong piece of evidence is to avoid peanuts (see page 181). The last trimester of pregnancy, the neo-natal period and the first week of life are cited as critical periods for allergic sensitization. Therefore, if exposure to highly allergenic foods can be avoided during these periods, the likelihood of your baby becoming allergic can be reduced or eliminated. If

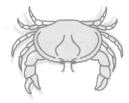

watch out!

Smoking during pregnancy can increase your child's chances of having allergies to food and other substances. In particular, smoking in early pregnancy appears to be most damaging. Children born in a household where one or more parents smoke are also more likely to develop allergies.

must know

Which probiotic?
Probiotic drinks are probably your best bet, as they are easily digested and easy to consume. High-probiotic yoghurts (these will have the number of healthy bacteria listed on the outside) are also good additions to your diet, and a great source of calcium and protein. Mix yoghurt with fresh fruit to create smoothies, or a little honey or ripe banana, which increases the probiotic (healthy bacteria) content. Otherwise, probiotic capsules are widely available. Keep them in the fridge, and take once or twice a day with food.

the baby's mother, father or a close relative has a history of severe allergies, it would be worth cutting down on the big eight – cow's milk, eggs, tree nuts, peanuts, soya, shellfish, fish and wheat products – certainly during the last three months of pregnancy and while breastfeeding. It is perfectly possible to have a healthy, balanced diet while keeping these particular foods to a minimum.

However, there is something positive a pregnant woman can do. A 2001 study found that women who take probiotics (acidophilus, for example), otherwise known as 'healthy' bacteria, during pregnancy can reduce the risk of their children becoming allergic, particularly if there is a family history of allergic illness. What is more, if a woman continues throughout breastfeeding (see opposite), the risk is reduced even further. The reasons why this appears to be successful is that it increases the amount of healthy bacteria in your child's body, which improves immunity, encourages a healthier digestive system and gut (which are implicated in many cases of food allergy), and may also help to create healthier enzymes in the gut, including lactase, which can prevent early lactose intolerance. Research into this is still ongoing, but it looks promising (see page 187). There is also some evidence that reducing the number of times a woman suffers from allergic reactions while she is pregnant can help reduce the chances of the baby becoming allergic. If a woman is reacting to allergens during pregnancy there is a high chance it will affect the baby and create a higher liklihood of the infant becoming allergic. So reducing allergens in the home and in the diet can make a difference.

Breastfeeding

In Chapter Five we looked at the benefits of breastfeeding in some detail, both as a preventative measure against allergies, and as the optimum source of nutrition for a baby. There are still other reasons why breastfeeding can help to prevent allergies and to keep your baby healthy.

The earlier and more often a food is eaten, the greater likelihood it has of becoming an allergen. Babies tend to be most allergic to the foods they have been offered first. When a baby is exclusively breastfed, he is only exposed to the foods his mother eats and secretes in her milk, so his exposure to potential allergens is minimized.

One long-term study of children who were breastfed showed that breastfeeding reduces food allergies at least through adolescence. For example, a 1994 study found that the incidence of cow's milk allergies is up to seven times greater in babies who are fed artificial baby milk instead of human milk.

Breastfeeding protects against allergies in two ways. The first and most obvious reason breastfed babies have fewer allergies is that they are exposed to fewer allergens in the first months of life. They aren't given formula-based cow's milk or soya products. Less exposure to these foods means less chance of allergy later on. The other reason breastfed babies have fewer allergies has to do with the development of the immune system. At birth, a baby's immune system is immature. Babies depend heavily on antibodies obtained from their mothers while in the womb. Their digestive systems are not

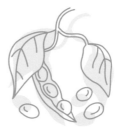

must know

Protection
There is also evidence that wheezing diseases, such as asthma, and other allergies, can be partially protected against when babies are breastfed. This has been backed up by no fewer than eight studies.

must know

Breastfeeding
Exclusive breastfeeding
(that is, to say, without
supplementing formula
or solid foods) is
required to sustain the
full benefits of allergy
protection. Although
partially breastfed
babies may be offered
some protection, the
introduction of
allergens through other
milks or foods can
hamper the process.
Aim to give exclusive
breastfeeding for at
least the first six
months of life.

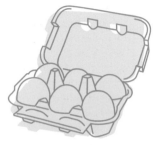

really ready for substances other than their mother's
milk. At about six weeks of age, Pyer's Patches in the
intestines begin to produce immunoglobulins or
antibodies. At six months of age, a baby has a
functional, if immature, immune system that is
capable of producing secretory immunoglobulin A
(sIgA), the antibody found in all body secretions that
is the first line of defence against foreign
substances. Look out for changes in feeding
patterns. A baby may show a marked dislike for milk
that contains foods to which he is allergic, or
become more drowsy when feeding after you have
eaten suspect foods. If a baby resists the breast, it is
worth looking at what you have recently consumed.
The La Lèche League confirms that allergenic foods
are not present in a mother's breast milk from about
seven days after removing it from the diet; therefore,
you should notice fairly quickly if you have found the
offending food. A baby's gut will allow allergenic
proteins across the wall until he is four to six
months old (see page 183), so a mother who is
breastfeeding a child at risk of a food allergy should
exclude allergenic foods (the 'big eight') until the
baby is at least four to six months of age.

In the meantime, a baby depends on mother's
milk for protection. Fed from his mother's breast, a
baby first receives colostrum, the first milk, which is
especially rich in antibodies, including sIgA. The sIgA
'paints' a protective coating on the inside of a baby's
intestines to prevent penetration by potential
allergens. Mature milk continues to provide this
protection from the inside to help the baby remain
healthy and allergy-free.

Diet and breastfeeding

Experts recommend that you breastfeed exclusively for six months in order for your baby to be given the best chance of avoiding allergies. But the duration is not only important, what you eat is also crucial.

Researchers do not recommend that breast-feeding mothers eliminate possible allergens from their diet if there is no family history of allergy, and the child is not showing signs of sensitivity. However, for an infant with an allergy or a family history, it is advisable to avoid the allergen during breastfeeding, as trace amounts of proteins that cause food allergies (such as those in milk, eggs, wheat and peanuts) can be transferred to a baby in breast milk.

Early and occasional exposure to proteins can sensitize a baby so that even small amounts may trigger a response: IgE levels rise and a severe reaction may occur. So even the tiny quantities that find their way to the baby through breast milk, or the odd bottle of formula, for example, can cause problems (if cow's milk is the allergen in question).

Look out for the signs

Remember, you do not need to suffer from a food allergy yourself for your baby to develop one, so it is important to watch for signs of allergy in your baby. If you are eating normally, and including all foods that might spark a reaction, and your baby is healthy, sleeping well, his skin is clear, and there are no bouts of unexplained crying or vomiting, it is unlikely that there is any real problem. However, some mothers find that their children suffer from eczema at a very young age, or vomit after their

must know

Milk proteins
Protein turnover takes at least four weeks. Therefore, the allergenic proteins in your diet will be in your breast milk for up to four weeks after you change your diet. Exclusion diets for women with a family history of food allergies should ideally begin at least four to six weeks before your baby's expected date of delivery.

mother has eaten large quantities of egg or dairy produce, for example. Keep a diary of what you eat, and make a note of any reactions.

Over time, it is usually possible to see connections between certain foods and a baby's distress. If highly allergic, a baby can react to foods their mother has eaten within minutes, although symptoms generally show up between four and 24 hours after exposure. You can develop an eating plan for yourself that eliminates suspect foods. If your baby seems happier, challenge your findings by eating some of the suspected food. A repeated reaction from your baby confirms his sensitivity, and you may well choose to limit or avoid the food for some time. It is, however, extremely important that breastfeeding mothers obtain the equivalent nutrients from other sources when excluding food groups – particularly milk (see page 132). Your dietitian or nutritionist can help you with this.

When a baby exhibits signs of food allergy while being exclusively breastfed (see page 180), you should keep an exposure diary to determine which foods in your diet might be implicated. Anything that seems to cause problems (gas, colic, mucus or blood in the stool, crying, eczema, etc.) in your baby should then be tested by an elimination diet, and then challenged under supervision. This, of course, means changing what *you* eat to see if it has any impact on symptoms. When the culprit foods have been identified, they should be excluded from your diet for the remainder of the time you breastfeed.

must know

Hidden allergens
Watch out for hidden sources of foods that may cause a reaction. For example, many breast creams and ointments contain peanut oil (arachnis oil), which can cause a reaction in susceptible babies.

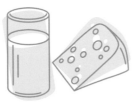

First foods

Your baby's diet in the first year of life is also extremely important for allergy prevention. In Chapter Five we looked at how and when to introduce solid foods. Let's look at why this is necessary.

First of all, it is never recommended that you begin weaning your baby before six months of age. Quite apart from allergies, there are other reasons for this. One of the most important reasons to avoid weaning before six months is because the digestive system – literally, from top to bottom – is immature and cannot cope with the addition of supplementary foods. For one thing, digestive enzymes develop slowly, first able to digest proteins at around three months of age, and then carbohydrates between the ages of 12 and 18 months. Nutrients are also more efficiently absorbed by the intestines as your baby grows older. Breast milk (and formula) are much more easily digested and absorbed by the body, and breast milk also contains enzymes that help to digest other foods, which is why it is important to keep up milk intake while you are weaning.

Secondly, a baby's gut is very porous and the lining only 'closes' properly around four or five months of age. Before this 'closure', large molecules of food and other substances are able to escape into the bloodstream, causing the body to recognize them as invaders and begin an immune response. This is significant because in susceptible children, it may result in an allergic response in the skin, lungs or gut. For example, children who are susceptible to coeliac disease (see page 154) may acquire the condition earlier if they receive foods containing gluten early in life.

Some studies show that early weaning may well be the cause of many food allergies and sensitivities in children. In fact, in 60 to 70 per cent of babies and young children who suffer from chronic diarrhoea, food sensitivities are at the root of the problem. And a study from Scotland found that persistent coughs, respiratory illness and eczema were more common in babies who had been given solid food before twelve weeks, than in those who were introduced to solids at a later stage.

Experts advise that you give your child one new solid food at a time, and to follow a certain sequence when introducing solids. The British Dietetic Association recommends beginning with traditional low-allergenic foods, such as rice, potatoes, root and green vegetables, apples, pears, bananas and stone fruit. Each new food should be tried on its own for a number of days before combining it with others, so that allergic triggers can be easily identified.

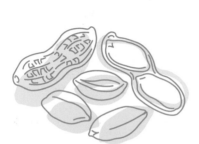

did you know?

Many children will resist solid foods if they contain allergens; this appears to be a defence mechanism, which creates a natural aversion to problem foods. Obviously all children need to eat some solid foods, but do not push foods that your child strongly resists. You do need to try out the top allergenic foods (apart from peanuts) by 12 months (see page 132), but if your child shows a repeated aversion, make a note of this and leave it for now. Avoiding problematic foods for at least the first year of life can increase the chances that your child will outgrow her an allergy or avoid one altogether.

Probiotics

We looked briefly at probiotics on page 180, and outlined the role they may play during pregnancy, by helping to prevent allergies. Although probiotics represent an exciting new area of research, there are still many gaps in our knowledge. For the time being, however, the results of a number of studies are promising.

Probiotic bacteria benefits

A large body of evidence over the past 75 years has demonstrated the preventive health value of eating foods fermented with Lactobacilli or Bifidobacteria. These beneficial bacteria are referred to as 'probiotics'. Probiotic bacteria are considered 'friendly' bacteria. They are an essential component of a healthy gastrointestinal tract as they inhibit the growth of harmful bacteria, boost immune function, decrease infection in the digestive tract, and enhance digestion through enzyme production. Some foods have added probiotics as healthy nutritional ingredients and this will be evident on the label. Supplements are also available. However, it is worth noting that the impact of your probiotic depends on the quantity of bacteria, the type of bacteria and whether or not it is successfully carried through to the intestines where they work.

During the first days of life, bacteria within an infant's intestines begin sending signals to the immune system. Healthy bacteria in the digestive tract allow the immune system to mature properly. On the other hand, unhealthy, aggressive bacteria can programme the immune system in such a way that it responds in a hyper-allergic or hyper-

must know
Prebiotics
are non-digestible, naturally occurring carbohydrates that come from foods like tomatoes, bananas, onions or artichoke hearts. Like fibre, they help maintain a healthy digestive system. Prebiotics are also the 'food' for the friendly bacteria. They can be added to the diet to increase the chances of beneficial bacteria growing and thriving in the digestive system.

inflammatory manner. Studies published during the past few years demonstrate that supplementing infants with probiotics leads to a nearly 50 per cent reduction in allergic illnesses like eczema – a reduction that persists throughout at least the first four years of life. Breastfeeding mothers can pass on the benefits by taking probiotics themselves; also when your baby is old enough, the contents of probiotic capsules can be sprinkled into purées or juice.

Most parents do not realize how often baby's eczema is triggered by food allergies – indeed, how often it is the first sign of food allergies. In one study, about 40 per cent of babies with eczema had proven food allergies. And the worse the rash, the more likely there is a food allergy involved. For the third of babies with the worst eczema, more than 96 per cent have a proven food allergy connection. Babies with eczema often have different ratios of beneficial bacteria in their guts, compared with other healthy babies; this has led to speculation that these bacteria are part of the allergy-eczema link.

In an April 2005 study, researchers investigated whether giving babies probiotics (beneficial bacteria) could improve their eczema. There were 230 babies in the study, ranging in age from six weeks to just under one year old. All of the babies in the study were suspected of having a cow's milk allergy. All of the babies were switched to cow's-milk-free diets (and their breastfeeding mothers to cow's-milk-free diets). All of the babies were treated with topical medicines. Some of the babies also received daily supplements of probiotics; the rest received placebo capsules. All babies in the study improved, by an average of 65 per cent. But those babies with either a positive skin test or blood test for food allergy enjoyed a 32 per cent greater improvement if they got the probiotic Lactobacillus GG (LGG) supplement than if they got the placebo capsules. A study in mice (in whom egg allergies were induced) found that giving probiotics suppressed their allergic response. Studies still need to be performed in humans to see if this effect is mimicked.

So all round, it is worth considering probiotics for you and your child, as the benefits appear to be positive, and there are no known side effects. Breastfeeding mothers can take probiotics, which will pass through their milk; bottle-fed babies can be given a formula with probiotics added. You can add probiotics to your baby's diet when you begin weaning. There are a variety of different forms now available, including probiotic drinks, although these should not be offered to young babies until about 12 months of age, as they usually contain cow's milk. Chewable tablets, or the contents of a capsule, sprinkled over food or into drinks, are good forms for older babies.

want to know more?

For help with breastfeeding an allergic baby, contact the La Lèche League. They have a 24-hour helpline (0845 120 2918), as well as a good website with plenty of information and advice. Visit www.laleche.org.uk.

Weaning an allergic baby can be difficult; there is plenty of helpful advice available at www.helpfoodallergy.com, or if your baby is allergic or sensitive to milk, visit www.milkfree.org.uk, which offers recipes and shopping tips as well. A Canadian organization, www.milkallergy.ca is also extremely useful.

Food can make you ill has information and resources on food intolerance. Visit www.foodcanmakeyouill.co.uk.

Allergy UK offers sound advice, information and support, and publishes details of clinics and specialists, plus local support groups. Helpline is 01322 619898 or visit www.allergyuk.org.

Want to know more?

Further reading

Hidden Food Allergies, Patrick Holford & Dr James Braly (Piatkus Books, 2006)

Allergy-free Cooking for Kids, Antoinette Savill, with Karen Sullivan (Thorsons, 2003)

The Complete Guide to Food Allergy and Intolerance, Jonathan Brostoff & Linda Gamlin (Bloomsbury, 1998)

The Candida Albican Yeast-free Cookbook: How Good Nutrition Can Help Fight the Epidemic of Candida, Pat Connolly (Keats, 2000)

Was It Something You Ate?: Food Intolerance - What Causes It and How to Avoid It, John Emsley & Peter Fell (Oxford University Press Inc, USA, 2001)

Your Allergy-free Diet Plan for Babies and Children, Carolyn Humphries (Foulsham, 2003)

Curing Food Allergies, Alan Hunter (Ashgrove Publishing, 2000)

The New Allergy Diet: The Step-by-step Guide to Overcoming Food Intolerance, J.O. Hunter, et al (Vermilion, 2000)

The Whole Foods Allergy Cookbook: 200 Gourmet and Homestyle Recipes for the Food Allergic Family, Cybele Pascal (Vital Health Publishing, 2005)

Useful Addresses

Websites

Food Allergy & Anaphylaxis Network
Nonprofit organization devoted to educating the public about food allergies. www.foodallergy.org

Living Without
Supporting and educating readers with allergies and food and chemical sensitivities.
www.livingwithout.com

Allergic-Child
Advice for parents on practical, everyday living for the family of a severely food allergic child.
www.allergicchild.com

Food-allergy.org
Provides books and information on the causes, diagnosis, and treatment of food allergies.
www.food-allergy.org

FoodIntol.com
Educational and support community for those with food intolerances and allergies. www.foodintol.com

Go Dairy Free
Guide to dairy-free living, including product lists and fast-food restaurant information.
www.godairyfree.org

Allergy and Allergies Agency
Web-based allergy resource maintained by Dr Adrian Morris with in-depth information on most of the common allergies encountered in the UK.
www.allergy-network.co.uk

Support organizations

The British Dietetic Association
5th Floor, Charles House
148/9 Great Charles Street
Queensway
Birmingham B3 3HT
Tel: 0121 200 8080
www.bda.uk.com

Medic Alert Foundation
MedicAlert® is a registered charity providing a life-saving identification system to protect and save lives
1 Bridge Wharf
156 Caledonian Road
London N1 9UU
Tel: 0800 581420
www.medicalert.org.uk

Food Standards Agency
PO Box 30080
Hanible House
Elephant and Castle
London SE1 6YA
Consumer Helpline: 0345 573012
www.food.gov.uk

Chemical Free
Aims to make life more tolerable for those affected by Multiple Chemical Sensitivity and Multiple Food Intolerance.
29 Kipling Close
Hitchin
Hertfordshire SG4 0DU
www.chemicalfree.co.uk

The Wheat and Dairy Free Supermarket
Hall Farm Court
Ripe
Lewes
East Sussex BN8 6AY
www.wheatanddairyfree.com

Glossary

Allergen: A substance that your body perceives as dangerous and causes an allergic reaction.

Allergy: An exaggerated response to a substance or condition produced by the release of histamine or histamine-like substances.

Anaphylaxis: Severe, life-threatening allergic response that may include swelling, breathing difficulties, shock and hives.

Angioedema: Swelling similar to urticaria (hives), but the swelling occurs beneath the skin instead of on the surface.

Antibodies: Proteins that are produced by our immune system in order to protect our body from 'intruders' such as bacteria and viruses.

Antihistamine: Medication that prevents symptoms of congestion, sneezing and itchy, runny nose by blocking histamine receptors.

Asthma: A disease of the branches of the windpipe (bronchial tubes) that carry air in and out of the lungs. Asthma causes the airways to narrow, the lining of the airways to swell, and the cells in the airways to produce more mucus.

Atopy: A predisposition to develop allergy. Diagnosed by having at least one positive skin prick test response or personal or first degree family history of asthma, eczema or hay fever.

Bronchodilators: Medications used to relax the muscle bands that tighten around the airways during an asthma episode.

Casein: The principal protein of cheese.

Coeliac disease: An inflammatory disease of the intestine, possibly a delayed allergic reaction to gluten, found in wheat, rye, barley and oats.

Decongestant: Medication that shrinks swollen nasal tissues to relieve symptoms of nasal swelling, congestion and mucus secretion.

Dermatitis: Inflammation of the skin, either due to direct contact with an irritating substance or to an allergic reaction.

Dust mites: Microscopic insects that live in household dust and are common allergens. They live on dead skin cells and are found in mattresses, pillows, carpets, curtains and furniture.

Eczema: A group of skin conditions characterized by dry, red, flaky, itchy skin. The most common form of eczema is allergic or atopic eczema.

Elimination diet: A diet in which certain foods are temporarily discontinued from the diet to rule out the cause of allergy symptoms.

ELISA (enzyme-linked immunosorbent assay): Blood test used to identify the substances that are causing your allergy symptoms.

Epinepherine (adrenaline): A medication for anaphylaxis that raises blood pressure and heart rate back to normal levels.

EpiPen: A device used to inject epinephrine during an anaphylaxis attack.

Food challenge: Test carried out in hospital to identify suspected food allergens by giving traces of food concealed in capsules or broth.

Hay fever: Allergic reaction caused by the pollens of ragweed, grasses and other plants.

Histamine: A naturally occurring substance that is released by the immune system after being exposed to an allergen.

Hypoallergenic: Products formulated to contain the fewest possible allergens.

Immunoglobulin E (IgE): A type of antibody responsible for most allergic reactions.

Immunotherapy: A series of shots that help build up the immune system's tolerance to an allergen.

Mast cell: A type of white cell that is involved in the allergic reaction.

Pollen: A fine, powdery substance released by plants.

RAST (radioallergosorbent test): Blood test used to identify the substances that are causing allergy symptoms and to estimate a sensitivity.

Rhinitis: An inflammation of the nasal passageways, particularly with discharge.

Sensitization: Alteration of the responsiveness of the body to the presence of foreign substances.

Skin prick test: A test where a needle is used to scratch the skin with a small amount of allergen. A response can usually be seen within 15 to 20 minutes.

Urticaria (hives): Itchy, swollen, red bumps or patches on the skin that appear suddenly as a result of the body's adverse reaction to certain allergens.

Index

Action Against Allergy 21, 97
acupuncture 112–13
additives 15, 17, 70, 140, 144–7, 150–1, 162
age, and allergy onset 17, 76
albumin 38
alcohol 71
allergens 12, 16–17, 23–67
allergic reactions 16, 100
allergy specialists 75, 76
Allergy UK 21, 150, 173, 187
almonds 44
amaranth 121
anaemia 137
anaphylaxis 12, 16, 87, 173
  biphasic 101
  definition 101
  foods which trigger 34–5, 42, 44–5, 47–8, 53, 57, 63–4
  signs of 101, 103
  treatment 101–3, 105
Anisakis 51
anthroposophic lifestyle 19
anti-allergy medications 78, 80
anti-inflammatories 107
antibiotics 19, 78, 80, 160, 172
antibodies 12, 16, 180
antidepressants 14, 166
antihistamines 51, 78, 102, 104–6, 160
antispasmodics 166
applied kinesiology 93
arthritis 168
Asian food 15, 117, 119
asparagus 90
asthma 15, 19, 20, 76, 96, 106, 114, 161–3, 169, 179
  in children 145, 147, 161
  treatment 162–3
  triggers 25, 34, 37, 40, 57, 61–2, 66, 161–2
at-risk people 19–21
attention deficit hyperactivity disorder (ADHD) 146–7
autoimmune diseases 168
Ayurveda 115

babies
  allergy 26, 28, 31, 66–7, 76, 129, 130–4, 142–3
  milk for 26, 28, 31, 66, 134–8
  probiotics for 185–7
  weaning 138–41, 183–4, 187
baby foods, commercial 140
bacon 119
Baked asparagus risotto 90
bakeries 117
beclo-methasone 163
beef 127
benzoates 54
biopsies 154
bird-egg syndrome 34
blood tests 79–80, 82, 95–6, 154
Bolognese sauce 127
bowel symptoms 18
breastfeeding 36, 42, 52, 65, 130–1, 134–5, 142–3, 179–82, 187
bronchodilators 78, 106
buckwheat 56, 121
budesonide 163
buffets 117

caesarean section 130
caffeine 14, 17, 62–3, 71
calcium 29, 31, 53, 126
candida 60, 172
capsaicin 71
carmine 145
carob 121
Carrot and coriander soup 91
carrots 88, 91
case histories 76
case studies 66–7, 96–7, 151
casein 28, 29, 137
cheese 14
  substitutes 121, 127
chi 121
chicken 88, 90, 122–3, 125, 127
children 129–51
  allergic diseases of 154–5, 158–9, 161, 173, 186
  and allergy tests 78, 81, 96–7

and allergy treatment 105, 106
and elimination diets 83
outgrowing allergies 12, 20–1, 45, 97, 130–1
and specific allergy triggers 26–7, 33–5, 39–40, 43–5, 52, 65
  see also babies
chocolate 14, 17, 56, 64
Chocolate soda bread 126
chronic diseases 20
citrus fruit 14, 56, 62, 63
coeliac disease 13, 38–9, 65, 154–5, 183
coffee 56, 62–3
colic 134, 151
colostrum 135
colourings 145
complementary therapies 108–15
condiments 117
constipation 164–5
corn (maize) 20, 56–9, 121, 131
corticosteroids 107
cortisone 160
cradle cap 159
cravings 85
cross-contaminated food 48, 118
cytotoxic food testing (ALCAT) 94–5

defining food allergies 11–12, 15
dehydration 169
delayed pattern food allergy 147, 162
desensitization 94
diagnosing allergies 69–97, 112
diarrhoea 13, 18, 72, 101, 133–4, 147, 156, 184
  foods which trigger 25, 29, 34, 37, 39, 47, 51, 53, 57, 61, 63–4
  of irritable bowel syndrome 164, 167
dieticians 75, 85, 96–7
double-blind tests 81
dust mites 158, 160

ears 18
eating out 116–19
eczema 19, 20, 72, 76–7, 80, 96–7, 114, 131, 134, 147, 158–60, 184, 186
  foods which trigger 25, 28, 34–5, 37, 40, 57, 62–4, 66
  treatment 159–60
  types of 158–9
education 148–50
egg allergy 17, 32–5, 119, 130–1
egg substitutes 120
elimination diets 13, 26, 72–5, 82–91, 131, 181–2
  for allergic illnesses 162–3, 166
  for children 142–3
  recipes 88–91
  reintroduction 87
  simple 84–5
  strict 85–7
ELISA/ACT 95
emollients 160
emulsifiers 37
entertaining 118–19
epinephrine (adrenaline) 63, 105
EpiPen (epinephrine) 44, 47, 53, 57, 67, 102–5, 150
essential fatty acids (EFAs) 53, 135
ethnicity 26, 133, 156
evening primrose oil 160
exercise-induced food allergy 71
eyes 18

faintness 107
false negatives 79
fever-reducers 19
'few foods' diet 83, 85–7, 88–91
fibre 167
fish
  allergy 12, 17, 20, 50–3, 117, 119, 131
families 50
  nutritional qualities 31
flour substitutes 121
food aversion 11
food challenge tests 80–1
food diaries 72–3, 75–7, 100, 131–2, 142
food intolerances 6–7, 10–15, 40–1
food labels 104
food poisoning 70, 71

food sensitivity 10–11
fruit 90, 91, 126

gliadin 38, 154
globulin 38
gluten allergy/intolerance (coeliac disease) 13, 38–9, 41, 65, 154–5, 183
Gnocchi with sage and lemon sauce 124–5

hair analysis 93–4
Hamburgers 127
hay fever 19, 34, 71, 76, 94
headaches 13–15, 18, 63–4, 145, 147
healthy eating 84
helplines 21
herbal teas 86–7
herbalism 110–12, 114–15
heredity/atopy 19, 66, 130, 131, 176–8
hidden foods, allergenic 27, 30, 32–3, 36–7, 40–3, 46–9, 51, 53, 55, 57–61, 63, 65, 155
histamine 12, 14, 16, 78, 104–5
  non-allergic release 13, 51, 70–1
hives (urticaria) 13, 14, 15, 18, 72, 101, 107, 147, 171–3
  foods which trigger 28, 34, 37, 40, 44–5, 47, 51, 53, 57, 61–5
home-testing kits 92, 97
homeopathy 109–10
Honey roasted chicken and sweet potato 88
hydrogen breath test 157
hygienic lifestyles 163
hyperactivity 20, 146–7

immune system 12–13, 16, 86, 135, 181–2
immunoglobulin E (IgE) 16, 19, 28, 38, 40, 51, 77, 79, 82, 95, 113, 159, 162, 173
immunoglobulin G (IgG) 95
intestinal flora 26, 172
iridology 95
iron deficiency 137
irritable bowel syndrome (IBS) 20, 39, 164–7
Italian food 127

lactase deficiency 13, 25–7, 133–4, 156–7
lactase supplements 27, 65, 157
Lactobacillus acidophilus 167
lactose intolerance 13–14, 24–8, 65, 110, 133–4, 136–7, 156–7
lactose tolerance test 157
lamb 89, 91, 127
larynx 18
laxatives 166
lecithin 35, 36, 37
legumes (pulses) 36, 42, 44, 121
leucocytotoxic tests 95
life-long allergies 12
lungs 18

magnesium 40, 41
managing allergies 99–127
mast cells 16
medication, allergenic 27, 57, 70–1, 72–3
Medihaler-Epi 105
menstrual cycle 72
meridians 112
metabolic defects 13–14
migraine 14, 20, 57, 63–4, 169–70
milk
  cow's 13–14, 17, 24–31, 66, 96–7, 130–1, 133–7, 158, 179
  formula 66, 96–7, 133–4, 136, 142, 179
  goat's 24–5, 27, 137
  hydrolyzed formula 137, 142
  Lactofree 65
  sheep's 24–5, 27
  substitutes 121, 134, 136–7
  see also breastfeeding
minerals 114, 126
  see also multi-vitamin and minerals
MMR (measles, mumps, rubella) 19, 35
monoamine oxidase inhibitors (MAOs) 14
monosodium glutamate (MSG) 15, 144
Moroccan lamb and apricot tagine 89
mouths 18, 45
moxibustion 112

multi-vitamin and minerals 35, 41, 83, 143
multiple food allergies 66-7, 74-5
mustard 56, 64-5

Nambudriprad's Allergy Elimination Technique (NAET) 112
nausea 14, 25, 34, 40, 51, 53, 57, 63, 156
nose 18
nutritional supplements 114
nutritional therapies 113-14
Nutron test 95
nuts 12, 17, 46-7, 117
    see also peanuts

omega-3 fatty acids 53
oral allergy syndrome 71, 100
organic foods 40, 140

peanuts 12, 17, 42-5, 67, 117, 131, 176-7
pesticides 40, 84
pesto 127
pharmacological reactions 14-15
phyto-oestrogens 136-7
placebos 80-1
pollen 71
potentization 110
prana 115
prebiotics 185
pregnancy 42-3, 76, 130, 163, 176-9
preservatives 54, 60-2, 140
prevalence of food allergies 10, 20, 129
preventing food allergies 6, 175-87
probiotics 159, 160, 167, 178, 185-7
processed food 20, 52, 84
protein 36, 50, 57, 135, 181
    of cow's milk 24-5, 27-31, 133-6
    of eggs 32, 34
    sources 35, 37, 126
provocation-neutralization 94
psoriasis 170-1

quinoa 121, 126

RAST (radio-allergosorbent test) 47, 79-80, 95-6
recipes 65, 88-91, 120-7
rhinitis 15, 34, 40, 60, 64
risotto 90
Ritalin 146, 151

salbutamol 163
salicylates 145, 147, 151
sauces 124-5, 127
school 149-50
selenium 53
self-help 107
serotonin 14
sesame seeds 48-9, 56, 117
shellfish 12-13, 17, 52-5, 117, 131
Shepherd's pie 127
shock 61, 145
    see also anaphylaxis
sIgA 180
sinuses 18
skin 18, 82
    see also eczema; hives
skin prick tests 47, 64, 77-9, 80, 96
smoking 163, 177
soda bread, chocolate 126
sodium benzoate 15
sodium chromoglycate 163
soups 91
soya 17, 36-7, 121, 127, 131, 134, 136-7
staphylococci 158, 159
steroids 78, 102, 107, 160, 163
stomach symptoms 18
stool acidity test 157
sugar 146
sulphates 56, 60-2, 84, 144-5, 162
sulphur dioxide 61, 62
sweet potato 88, 89, 91, 125
Sweet potato, chickpea and parsley mash 125
symptoms, allergic 18, 76
    in children 131-2, 181-2
    chocolate allergy 65
    coffee allergy 63
    dairy allergy 28-9, 31, 34-5
    fish/shellfish allergy 51, 53-5

grain allergy 39-40, 57
mustard allergy 65
nut allergy 44-5, 47
soya allergy 37
sulphate allergy 61

tartrazine 15, 145
terbutaline 163
tests 12, 26, 75, 75-97, 82, 154, 157
    repeat 81
    see also elimination diet
Thai green chicken curry 122-3
Traditional Chinese Medicine (TCM) 114-15
treatment for allergies
    complementary 108-15
    emergency 103
    medical 101-3, 104-7
tryptamine 14
tyramine 14, 62

vaccinations 19, 34, 35
vasoactive amines 14-15
VEGA testing 92-3
vegetables, leafy green 31, 126
vitamin A 29, 31, 35, 53
vitamin B complex 29, 35, 40, 41
vitamin D 29, 31, 35, 53
vitamin E 29, 31, 35, 40
vitamins 114, 126
    see also multi-vitamin and minerals
vomiting 13, 18, 28-9, 34, 37, 39, 40, 47, 51, 57, 64, 72, 101, 134

weals 77-8
weaning 138-41, 183-4, 187
wet wraps 160
wheat allergy 17, 20, 38-41, 65, 151, 154-5
wheat substitutes 121
whey 28, 29
wine 14, 17

yeast 14, 15, 60
yoghurt 24, 27, 31, 121, 178

zinc 35, 40, 41